IF YOU'RE GOING TO BED,
YOU HAVE TO *PLAN* TO GO TO SLEEP.

Don't take a pre-sleep shower. It's a stimulant.
Do take a hot bath two hours before bedtime.

Don't read a horror novel.
Do read calming poetry or a short story.

Don't have a cigarette. It will cause an "alert calm."
Do try a banana milkshake.

Don't become obsessed with how late it is.
Do turn your alarm clock toward the wall.

Above all...

Don't worry,

and

Do have a good night, and pleasant dreams.

Seven Days to a Perfect Night's Sleep

Debra L. Gordon

St. Martin's Paperbacks

SEVEN DAYS TO A PERFECT NIGHT'S SLEEP

Copyright © 2003 by Lynn Sonberg.

Cover photo © Janis Christie/Getty.

ISBN: 0-312-98583-5

Printed in the United States of America

St. Martin's Press Griffin edition / April 2003
St. Martin's Paperbacks edition / April 2003

St. Martin's Paperbacks are published by St. Martin's Press, 175 Fifth Avenue, New York, NY 10010.

10 9 8 7 6 5 4 3 2 1

Author's Note

This book is for informational purposes only. It is not intended to take the place of medical advice from a trained medical professional. Readers are advised to consult a physician or other qualified health professional about all problems with sleep or other health concerns, and before making any substantial changes in their diet or adopting the suggestions in this book. The author, proprietor, and publisher disclaim any liability arising directly or indirectly from the use of this book.

The fact that an organization or Web site is listed in this book as a potential source of information does not mean that the author or publisher endorses any of the information it may provide or recommendations it may make.

Research about sleep and sleep disorders is ongoing and subject to conflicting interpretations and new information. Likewise, readers should be advised that Web sites offered as sources for further information may have changed since this was written.

Contents

Seven Days

to a

Perfect

Night's

Sleep

One

Desperately Seeking Sleep

By any measuring stick, the deaths, illness and damage due to sleep deprivation and sleep disorders represent a substantial problem for American society.
   —from "Wake Up America: A National Sleep Alert,"
   1993 Report of the National Commission on Sleep
   Disorders Research

IT IS PAST 11 P.M., AND MY CAT, DOG, CHILDREN, AND husband are asleep around me in the eerily silent house. I promised myself an hour ago I would head for bed. I am feeling the effects of a long day that began at 6:30 and involved three hours of driving, many hours of computer work, overseeing homework, and dinner duty, with a myriad of decisions and tasks along the way. The stresses of the day have made my throat scratchy, the sign of an imminent cold.

Yet I want to get this chapter written. Giving up a few hours of sleep seems like a small price to pay for the satisfaction of meeting a deadline. I forge on and, like six out of ten Americans, I don't get enough of that precious commodity—sleep. This would be true even on nights when I do get to bed early, because like half of all Americans, I suffer from occasional insomnia.

That's where *Seven Days to a Perfect Night's Sleep* comes in.

By following this simple seven-day sleep program, you will be able to make the necessary adjustments to your environment, your presleep routine, your diet, and your exercise habits so you can get a sound night's sleep every night. Not every suggestion will work for you. Your insomnia is as individual as you are. But through trial and error you should be able to put together a program that will end your sleepless nights.

The Power of Sleep

In 1910, most Americans slept about nine hours per night. Today, one-third of us sleeps less than seven hours a night—far fewer than the eight or more hours that sleep experts recommend; three in ten are actually sleeping less than we did just five years ago. Physically and mentally we still require the same amount of sleep. We've just come to view sleep as expendable in the busyness of our lives.

According to the 2000 National Sleep Foundation (NSF) "Sleep in America" poll, we're spending more time at work and less time asleep than we did five years ago. The more we work, the NSF found, the more insomnia we experience. "This is particularly noticeable for people working more than 40 hours per week," says NSF vice-president James C. Walsh, Ph.D. Three out of ten of us work 50 hours or more per week.

We also live in an open-all-night society. These days, you can buy groceries, print your resumé, and bowl a perfect game—all at 3 a.m. in most cities. The global economy has many of us working at unusual hours: When it's midnight here, the stock markets are already in full swing in Japan. Finally, there are the scapegoats for most of modern society's ills—television and the Internet. In fact, four out of ten adults don't sleep because they're doing such things as watching *Survivor* or bidding on eBay.

Nearly half—45 percent—of all adults surveyed in the

NSF poll say they'll sleep less than eight hours to get more done for work, home, family, and hobbies. Even if we do get the optimum number of hours of sleep, our slumber is likely to be filled with disruption. Seven out of ten of us experience frequent sleep problems; more than 40 million Americans suffer from sleep disorders, most of them undiagnosed.

We can't fall asleep, stay asleep, or get the benefits that sleep promises. As a result, far too many of us go through our days in a haze, dozing in meetings, at the wheel, in front of the television after dinner. The NSF poll found that one in five adults is so sleepy during the day it interferes with daily activities. Yet we don't nap and we don't take breaks. We just keep going, trying to fight off the fatigue, often with dangerous or even fatal results as we sink farther and farther into sleep debt. Former President Bill Clinton once said that every big mistake he made in his life was because he was tired.

The world is waking up to the importance of sleep, helped by the field of sleep research, which didn't take hold in this country until the late 1960s. Research findings that adolescents function better when they can sleep later and start school later led to legislation in some towns requiring that schools open later. And studies showing the high numbers of accidents caused by sleep-deprived drivers resulted in at least one state's charging those drivers with vehicular homicide if their victim dies.

Sleep is no longer thought of as the space between the activities of our days. Today, researchers know that sleep contributes to every aspect of our well-being, from our immune system to our mental health.

Why Don't We Sleep?

Stress and anxiety are the most common reasons for insomnia, and in today's post-9/11 world, those two elements have risen to dangerous levels. Soon after the horrors of September 11, for instance, the number of Americans experiencing sleep problems skyrocketed. A poll by the National Sleep Foundation found that nearly half of respondents reported symptoms of insomnia as they tried to sleep in the nights immediately following the attacks, with nearly half having trouble falling asleep or staying asleep, or waking up feeling unrefreshed—all signs of insomnia. These problems did not just beset those in the Northeast. Researchers found no statistical difference by region in the quality of people's sleep.

Of course, it takes more than terrorism to cause our sleep problems. The simple stresses of everyday life—deadlines at work, marital problems, a fight with your teenager, worries over your job or finances—can all have you staring at the ceiling at 3 a.m. About one-fourth of adults report that "thinking about something" causes sleep problems. Stress and anxiety are the most common reasons for insomnia, and in today's post-9/11 world, those two elements have risen to dangerous levels. Further, the problems that keep them awake are related more often to personal issues (47 percent) than work issues (29 percent).

The High Cost of Sleeplessness

Three Mile Island, Chernobyl, *Exxon Valdez*, the space shuttle *Challenger*—each of these names brings to mind images of horrific disaster. Did you know each was related, at least in part, to sleep problems?

Overall, the National Commission on Sleep Disorders estimates that sleep-related accidents cost the American government $46 billion per year, while sleep disorders, sleep deprivation, and fatigue add another estimated $15.9 billion to the national healthcare bill. Fatigue even plays a role in nursing home statistics: Disturbed sleep is among the reasons most frequently cited by caretakers for institutionalizing older Americans.

But it is driving and fatigue where the greatest dangers lie. Thirty-one percent of commercial truck crashes that were fatal to the driver were caused by drowsiness. Sleepy drivers cause at least 100,000 police-reported crashes, 40,000 injuries, and 1,550 fatalities a year. Fall-asleep crashes may kill more young Americans than alcohol-related crashes.

That's because sleep deprivation and driving don't mix, particularly if you're driving between 2 and 4 p.m., when your natural sleep/wake cycles dip. Drowsiness slows reaction time, decreases awareness, and impairs your judgment, all of which lead to traffic accidents.

"We are facing enormous public safety consequences," says National Sleep Foundation executive director Richard L. Gelula. "We have more vehicles and more drivers driving more miles each year, and a huge number of them are literally asleep at the wheel. This cannot be ignored as an unfortunate consequence of hectic, modern living."

The day may soon come when a cop pulls you over and, instead of administering a breathalyzer, gives you a sleep deprivation test.

Dozing Off at Work

In addition to physical danger, our growing sleep debt plays havoc with our performance in the workplace. According to a 2001 Sleep in America National Sleep Foundation poll, workers estimated that the output and the quality of their work declined about 30 percent when they were sleepy. Twenty-seven percent of those questioned said they were sleepy at work two or more days a week. Thirty-one percent of women said they were tired on the job, compared to 22 percent of men.

Nearly one in seven workers said they were occasionally or frequently late to work because of sleepiness. The younger the person, the more likely she or he is to be late, with 22 percent of those in the 18 to 29 age range saying they're late to work because of sleepiness.

Almost one in five workers said they occasionally or frequently made mistakes at work because of fatigue. The highest percentages were from those in sales (35 percent), retail (33 percent), and financial, insurance, and real estate professionals (29 percent). When they're tired on the job, workers reported, they have a harder time concentrating, handling stress, solving problems, and making decisions. They can't even listen to coworkers if they haven't had enough sleep.

You might want to ask your surgeon how much sleep he or she has gotten the next time you're in for surgery, especially if your doctor is still in training. Surgical residents often go 36 hours or more without sleep. After 24 hours without sleep, researchers find that motor performance is comparable to that of someone who is legally intoxicated.

Sleep and Your Health

Lack of sleep affects your health as much as it affects your performance. University of Chicago researchers found that sleep deprivation can lead to insulin resistance, a risk factor for diabetes. The researchers studied 27 healthy adults, 14 of whom were normal sleepers, and 13 of whom got less than five hours of sleep a night. Those who continually got too little sleep not only developed a sleep debt, but experienced disruptions in other body functions, which affected their overall health. In another study of 11 healthy young men, the researchers found that after only four hours of sleep for six consecutive nights the men's blood glucose levels nearly matched those of people with diabetes.

Military researchers found that too little sleep over an extended period of time can cause permanent brain damage. Even short-term sleep deprivation can be harmful. Anyone who's ever stayed up all night to cram for a test or to write a paper may have experienced the fuzziness and forgetfulness that often results the next day. The military studies found that even after four eight-hour nights of sleep, sleep-deprived subjects still made more errors than they did before they fell into sleep debt.

Other researchers found that not getting enough sleep results in higher levels of stress hormones the next morning, which may adversely affect your memory, your immune system, or even the health of your heart. Another study found that sleep deprivation can affect levels of thyroid hormones, critical to a variety of functions, including general energy level and metabolism.

We can't learn new tasks or remember information for a test if we don't get enough sleep, because sleep plays such a large role in memory. Too little sleep may even contribute to breast cancer because of its effect on levels of the sleep-related hormone melatonin. In studies, breast cancer cells incubated in alternating levels of melatonin—high for 12 hours, low for 12 hours—approximating normal melatonin cycles, were least likely to grow, suggesting that melatonin is part of a woman's inborn defense against breast cancer. This may explain why a 1991 study found that blind women were only half as likely to get breast cancer as sighted women. They were subjected to less light and therefore had higher levels of melatonin.

As for the more everyday effects of sleep on health, continually shortchanging your sleep time lowers your immunity to colds or the flu. In studies, a rat kept awake for two weeks will die of infection because its immune system is simply too worn out to function. If humans persistently get less sleep than needed, the risk of dying prematurely is 70 percent higher than those who get enough sleep.

Lack of sleep can contribute to weight gain. One week of sleep deprivation can reduce production of a growth hormone that helps control the body's proportion of muscle to fat, a factor important in controlling body weight. If you don't produce enough of this hormone, you tend to store fat. Too little sleep also reduces levels of leptin, a hormone that plays a huge role in your ability to control how much you eat, causing carbohydrate cravings even when you feel full. Unless you burn those excess calories, unlikely because fatigue can reduce your desire to work out, they'll be converted to body fat.

Sleep and Your Emotions

Marsha Shapiro, a 35-year-old mother of three from Atlanta, describes her mood when she gets less than eight hours of sleep: "Grumpy, no patience with my kids, shaky, can't focus, short-tempered." This is the power of sleep.

Even the ancients understood the importance of a good night's sleep. As the rabbis said in the Talmud, "He that stays awake at night imperils his own life."

For years, freelance photographer and writer Liz Reap went through periods she thought were depression. "I'd start thinking extremely negatively about myself, the world around me, problems I need to solve, even people I love," recalls Reap, who lives in Kutztown, Pennsylvania. "I'd get really sad and hopeless, overwhelmed about things like laundry, scheduling issues, and feel really fatigued."

Reap began to notice a pattern. The moods overtook her right after she'd finished some kind of "work marathon," in which she forced herself to stay up late for several days in a row to meet her deadlines, or after her body experienced a time change, as when she traveled cross-country.

"Sure enough, I'd reach a point where my body would just shut down, then I'd end up sleeping for 14 to 16 hours," Reap recalls. "But after I started to understand what rest and sleep does for you, it was like waking up in the middle of a laundry detergent commercial. Birds are chirping, flowers are blooming, and my eyes are no longer squinting from trying so hard to concentrate. Headache gone, backache gone. The most important change I noticed, though, was my ability to focus. Without enough rest, I find that my mind wanders . . . but if I get enough sleep, I'm able to concentrate much longer."

Today, she says, sleep has become one of her favorite activities. "I never thought I'd say this, but I'd much rather go to bed at 9 p.m. than stay up to watch late-night TV anymore." She now views sleep the same way she views eating. "When my tank runs out, I've found that sleep—at times more than eating—is the best way to regain physical well-being and mental clarity."

Counting Your Sleep Debt

Most of us have pulled "all-nighters" at one time or another. It may have been in college, staying up with a sick child, finishing that report due at 10 a.m., or simply frantically cleaning the house and cooking for a last-minute visit from relatives—whatever the reason, sleep is often viewed as dispensable in times of need.

Thus, most of us owe more to the sleep bank than to our mortgage companies. For sleep debt—whether it is 5 hours or 500 hours—is a very real phenomenon, one whose interest can be just as deadly as that owed to a loan shark. Eventually, that loan comes due.

No matter how long you put it off, at some point you must pay back accumulated sleep debt. Sleep literature is filled with stories of researchers who didn't realize how sleep-deprived they were until they went on vacation and slept nearly around-the-clock for two days. In one study from the National Institute of Mental Health, healthy young volunteers spent 14 hours in bed in the dark. During the first few days, they slept about 11 hours a night. That amount dropped during the following three weeks, as they paid back their sleep debt—about 17 hours. By the fourth week of the experiment, the volunteers slept an average of 8 hours and 15 minutes a night. They had finally moved their sleep account into the black.

Sleep deprivation is cumulative. There is no way you ever "get used to it," and it will not go away over time unless you sleep it off. It doesn't take much to make you feel off your mark. Burning eyes, fuzzy brain, irritability—even a sense of feeling cold or craving high-fat foods can be attributed to as little as seven or eight hours of sleep debt.

The deeper in debt you are, the more devastating the effects. Labor mediators, for example, often deliberately build up a sleep debt in their clients on both sides to make use of the fuzzy thinking and sloppiness that goes along with exhaustion, knowing it will be easier to bring the two parties to an agreement by the final deadline. As one mediator told Stanley Coren in his book *Sleep Thieves* (Free Press, 1996), "No matter how far apart the parties are at the start of the [negotiation] process, if they get tired enough they'll find some compromise so that they can end the discussion and go home to sleep."

Sleep debt may begin with skipping a few hours of sleep, and it builds from there. A night of interrupted sleep, poor sleep, or simply setting the alarm to get up too early can add to the imbalance. One study found that reducing the amount you sleep as little as 1.3 to 1.5 hours for one night results in reduction of daytime alertness by as much as 32 percent. Overall, an October 16, 2000 *U.S. News and World Report* article estimated that by the end of the year, most Americans are short 338 hours—two full weeks—of sleep.

How Sleepy Are You?

To determine how tired you really are, complete the following questionnaire, which will help you measure general levels of daytime fatigue. Answers are rated on a scale called the Epworth Sleepiness Scale (ESS). This is the same tool sleep experts use.

Each item describes a routine daytime situation. Mark the answer that best describes the likelihood that you would doze off or fall asleep during that activity.

0 = would never doze
1 = slight chance of dozing
2 = moderate chance of dozing
3 = high chance of dozing

Situation	Chance of Dozing (0–3)
Sitting and reading	
Watching television	
Sitting inactive in a public place such as a theater or meeting	
Sitting as a passenger in a car for an hour without a break	
Lying down to rest in the afternoon	
Sitting and talking to someone	
Sitting quietly after lunch (when you've had no alcohol)	
Sitting in a car while stopped in traffic	

Evaluate your total score:
0–5: Slight or no sleep debt
5–10: Moderate sleep debt
11–20: Heavy sleep debt
20 or above: Extreme sleep debt

To figure your own sleep debt on a given day or week, consider the average nightly amount of sleep you need. If it's eight hours, and you get just five hours a night during the work week, by Saturday you'll have a sleep debt of 15 hours.

As the Epworth Sleepiness Scale shows, the bigger your sleep debt, the stronger your tendency to fall asleep. When you doze during a long meeting, while in a warm room, or when riding in a car, it's not because the activities or surroundings themselves are sleep-inducing, but because you're so sleep-deprived that your body will take any "down" time as an opportunity to fall asleep.

Sleep debt also plays havoc with your reaction time, making it nearly as bad as or worse than the effects of alcohol. One study found that 20 to 25 hours of wakefulness had the same effect on performance as a blood alcohol level of 0.05 to 0.10. Even moderate levels of fatigue decreased performance, mimicking levels of alcohol intoxication that would be deemed unacceptable when driving, working, or operating dangerous equipment.

The Seven-Day Sleep Program

This book presents a seven-day program that will help you pay your sleep debt. Paying back the sleep bank will provide you with a newfound energy and vitality that will be reflected in every aspect of your life.

In each day of the program, we'll tackle a different cause of insomnia and I'll offer tips and recommendations for dealing with it. Then we'll combine these strategies into a comprehensive sleep approach, until, by the end of the week, you should be sleeping as soundly as a bear in January.

Before you begin in the program you need to map your sleep habits by completing a sleep diary, explained in Chapter 3. In addition, if your insomnia is chronic, you should visit your doctor to rule out any possible medical conditions. As you'll see in chapters 5 and 6, there are dozens of sleep-related and other physical conditions that can interfere with a good night's sleep, as well as numerous treatments to resolve them and improve your sleep.

Simply learning all you can about effective sleep habits, whether you put them into use or not, can help you sleep better. One study found that increasing participants' knowledge about sleep patterns enabled most to go from 60 minutes of wakefulness a night to less than 30. So, in Chapter 2 we'll spend a little time learning about sleep.

How Sleep-Smart Are You?

Take the following quiz. The correct answers are below.

1. Sleep is a time when your body and brain shut down for rest and relaxation.
   True_____False_____

2. If you regularly doze off unintentionally during the day, you may need more than just a good night's sleep.
   True_____False_____

3. If you snore loudly and persistently at night and are sleepy during the day, you may have a sleep disorder.
   True_____False_____

4. Opening the car window or turning the radio up will keep the drowsy driver awake.
   True_____False_____

5. Narcolepsy is a sleep disorder marked by "sleep attacks."
   True_____False_____

6. The primary cause of insomnia is worry.
   True_____False_____

7. One cause of not getting enough sleep is restless legs syndrome.
   True_____False_____

8. The body has a natural ability to adjust to different sleep schedules such as working different shifts or traveling through multiple time zones quickly.
True_____ False_____

9. People need less sleep as they grow older.
True_____ False_____

10. More people doze off at the wheel of a car in the early morning or midafternoon than in the evening.
True_____ False_____

ANSWERS:

1. **False.** Although sleep is a time when your body rests and restores its energy levels, sleep is an active state that affects both your physical and mental well-being. Adequate restful sleep, like diet and exercise, is critical to good health. Insufficient restful sleep can result in mental and physical health problems and possibly premature death.

2. **True.** Many people doze off unintentionally during the day despite getting their usual night's sleep. This could be a sign of a sleep disorder. Approximately 40 million Americans suffer from sleep disorders, including sleep apnea, insomnia, narcolepsy, and restless legs syndrome. An untreated sleep disorder can reduce your daytime productivity, increase your risk of accidents, and put you at risk for illness and even early death.

3. **True** Persistent loud snoring at night and daytime fatigue are the main symptoms of a common and serious sleep disorder, sleep apnea. Another symptom is frequent long pauses in breathing during sleep, followed by choking and gasping for breath. People with sleep apnea don't get enough restful sleep, and their daytime performance is

often seriously affected. Sleep apnea may also lead to hypertension, heart disease, heart attack, and stroke. However, it can be treated, and the sleep apnea patient can live a normal life.

4. **False.** Opening the car window or turning the radio up may rouse a sleepy driver briefly, but this won't keep that person alert behind the wheel. Even mild drowsiness is enough to reduce concentration and reaction time. The sleep-deprived driver may nod off for a couple of seconds at a time without even knowing it—enough time to kill him/herself or someone else. This condition has been responsible for an average of 56,000 reported accidents each year—claiming over 1,500 lives.

5. **True.** People with narcolepsy fall asleep at any time of the day and in all situations, regardless of the amount or quality of sleep they've had the night before. Narcolepsy is characterized by "sleep attacks," as well as by daytime fatigue, episodes of muscle weakness or paralysis, and disrupted nighttime sleep. Although there is no known cure, medications and behavioral treatments can control symptoms, and people with narcolepsy can live normal lives.

6. **False.** Insomnia has many different causes, including physical or mental conditions and stress. Insomnia is a condition in which you don't get enough sleep because you can't fall asleep, stay asleep, or get back to sleep once you've awakened during the night. It affects people of all ages, usually for just an occasional night or two, but sometimes for weeks, months, or even years. Because insomnia can become a chronic problem, it is important to get it diagnosed and treated if it persists for more than a month.

7. **True.** Restless legs syndrome (RLS) is a medical condition distinguished by tingling sensations in the legs—and sometimes the arms—while sitting or lying still, especially at bedtime. The person with RLS constantly needs to stretch or move the legs to try to relieve these uncomfortable or painful symptoms. As a result, he or she has difficulty falling asleep or staying asleep and usually feels extremely tired and unable to function fully during the day. Good sleep habits and medication can help the person with RLS.

8. **False.** Our biological clock programs us to feel sleepy at night and to be active during the day. People who work the night shift and try to sleep during the day are constantly fighting their biological clocks. This puts them at risk of error and accident at work and of disturbed sleep. The same is true for people who travel through multiple time zones quickly; they get "jet lag" because they cannot maintain a regular sleep/wake schedule. Sleeping during the day in a dark, quiet bedroom and getting exposure to sufficient bright light at the right time can help improve daytime alertness.

9. **False.** As we get older, we don't need less sleep, but we often get less sleep. Our ability to sleep for long periods and to get into the deep restful stages of sleep decreases with age. Older people experience a more fragile sleep and are more easily disturbed by light, noise, and pain. They also may have medical conditions that contribute to sleep problems. Going to bed at the same time every night and getting up at the same time every morning, getting exposure to natural outdoor light during the day, and sleeping in a cool, dark, quiet place at night may help.

10. **True.** Our bodies are programmed by our biological clock to experience two natural periods of sleepiness during the

24-hour day, regardless of the amount of sleep we've had in the previous 24 hours. The primary period is between about midnight and 7:00 a.m. A second period of less intense sleepiness is in the midafternoon, between about 1:00 and 3:00. This means that we are more at risk of falling asleep at the wheel at these times than in the evening—especially if we haven't been getting enough sleep.

[Source: National Heart, Lung and Blood Institute.]

Two

Understanding This Thing We Call Sleep

THE SCIENCE OF SLEEP IS RELATIVELY YOUNG. IT IS ONLY in the past 40 years that researchers have delved into its mysteries, helped along by a variety of technologies that measure brain waves, how the heart reacts, and other physiological states.

They've learned that rather than being one long session, sleep is actually composed of several distinct stages. And that the mechanisms of sleep are governed by a complex interaction between light and darkness, body temperature, hormone release, and your own genetic background. Understanding sleep will, in turn, help you find a better night's sleep for yourself.

Circadian Rhythms

Are you a lark or a night owl? In sleep parlance, larks are morning people, those who bound out of bed and face the world with a smile even before the first cup of coffee. Night owls, on the other hand, don't start waking up until noon, regardless of how early they have arisen, and find it difficult to wind down before midnight. In general, more women are larks and more men are owls. (This may, of course, have something to do with who gets up to take care of the kids.) And, notes sleep researcher James B. Maas, Ph.D., in his book *Power Sleep* (Villard Books, 1998), when larks and owls marry, they spend less time in serious conversations and shared activities, including sex, than those who share similar wake/sleep cycles.

Consider the schedule Connecticut couple Donna and Ray follow. Both avowed night owls, they sleep from 4 a.m. to noon, then work (she as a freelance writer, he as an electronic engineer at a television station) from 3 p.m. to midnight. They exercise, eat "dinner" around 1 a.m., run errands (the 24-hour grocery store is a lifesaver), then do housework or just relax until it's time for bed at 4 a.m.

Compare them to Cherry Key Glogg, an assignment editor for a New York City television station, who calls herself a morning person. Her mornings start at 3 a.m., when she gets up to go to work, which she doesn't mind in the least. "Generally I'm wide awake and ready to go," she says of her early rising time. She usually doesn't need an alarm to wake up, a sign she's getting enough sleep. She's kept this schedule through two pregnancies, and finds it works well with children, since she's home in the early afternoon for homework, sports, etc. And she rarely has trouble falling asleep at night, around 8 p.m., when her three-year-old son also goes to bed. Friday afternoons and evenings are the most difficult, she says. "By that time, I'm really tired and cranky." To compensate, she sleeps late (for her) on weekends—until 7 a.m.

Donna and Ray, on the other hand, have followed their night owl schedule for two years, yet still don't sleep well and often suffer bouts of insomnia. The reason? They're playing "sleep roulette" with their circadian rhythms, a complex ballet of temperature cycles and hormones that create an inner clock that regulates your sleep/wake cycles. This powerful clock is activated even before birth, when a mother passes on her rhythms to her fetus. Sleep researcher William C. Dement, M.D., Ph.D., suggests a mother's circadian rhythm acts as a "gatekeeper," preventing birth from occurring during the day. Most mammals, he notes in his book *The Promise of Sleep* (Dell, 1999), give birth when they would normally tend to be asleep, "perhaps to make sure the birth happens at home, and thus safe from predators."

The term "circadian" comes from the Latin words "circa dies," meaning, "about a day." Every living thing—including plants—experiences some form of circadian rhythm. One would expect our inner clock to run on a 24-hour cycle, but it doesn't. When researchers put volunteers into isolation with few visual or social clues, they discovered that humans run on about a 25-hour clock.

The "clock" that governs these rhythms, called the suprachiasmatic nucleus or SCN, is actually a pair of pinhead-sized brain structures that together contain about 20,000 neurons. It rests in the part of the brain called the hypothalamus, just above the point where the optic nerves cross. The SCN governs body functions that affect and are affected by the sleep/wake cycle, including temperature, hormone secretion, urine production, and changes in blood pressure. It may even play a role in disease. Strokes and asthma attacks tend to occur more frequently during the night and early morning, perhaps due to changes in hormones, heart rate, and other characteristics associated with sleep.

Light that reaches photoreceptors in the retina (a tissue at the back of the eye) creates signals that travel along the optic nerve to the SCN. Then, signals from the SCN travel to several brain regions, including the pineal gland, which responds to these light-induced signals by switching off production of the hormone melatonin. This is what wakes us up.

As the day progresses, and light fades, the pineal gland receives a signal to increase production of the hormone melatonin, getting us ready for bed. This complex arrangement of light and melatonin may be one reason we tend to be sleepier in the winter: As the number of daylight hours decreases and the brain secretes more melatonin, it's harder to wake up in the morning, and midafternoon naps become more tempting.

The melatonin/light relationship is the reason why many totally blind people experience lifelong sleeping problems. Because their retinas are unable to detect light, their circadian rhythms follow their innate—25-hour—cycle rather than a 24-hour one, leading to a feeling of permanent jet lag and periodic insomnia.

The Hormonal Sleep Cycle

Other hormones play a role in sleep beside melatonin. One of the most important is serotonin, the precursor to melatonin. Growth hormone (gH) is secreted primarily during the early phases of sleep. When we're young, gH is critical for growth; as we age, it plays an important role in repairing and regenerating tissue. Then, toward morning, as melatonin levels drop, levels of cortisol (a hormone that signals alertness) rise, peaking just when we awaken.

Female sex hormones also play a role, and may be one reason women generally have more sleep problems and more deep sleep than men, notes Joyce Walsleben, Ph.D., director of the sleep disorders center at NYU School of Medicine and author of *A Woman's Guide to Sleep* (Three Rivers Press, 2000). The female hormone progesterone seems to have a sedating effect (and is highest just before women menstruate, which may explain some of the fatigue of PMS), while estrogen seems to enhance REM sleep, which may explain the unusually vivid dreams many women say they have during pregnancy, when estrogen levels are higher.

Body Temperature

Although melatonin is called the "sleep hormone," it's still not clear exactly how it works to bring on sleep. One thing that is known, however, is that the melatonin/sleep interaction is dependent on temperature changes. Scientists have known for more than a century that our temperature changes throughout a 24-hour period, rising during the day and falling at night (about one degree). As temperature drops, melatonin levels rise—with the greatest rise taking place between 9 p.m. and midnight (when most of us go to sleep). Studies have found that melatonin itself directly affects that temperature drop. Taking supplemental melatonin during the day results in a temperature drop. This may be why taking a hot bath a couple of hours before bed helps you sleep: The rise in body temperature from the heat sends a signal to your body to release more melatonin to lower your body temperature—ergo, preparing you for sleep.

Zeitgebers

Everything from the party you're planning to attend tonight to the 8:15 train you have to catch in the morning affects your natural circadian rhythms. These external factors, including sunlight, social interactions, even outside noise (such as the early morning garbage truck or your alarm clock), are called zeitgebers (from the German words meaning "time givers"). These factors keep your internal clock synchronized with the external world. Even as those circadian rhythms push you toward a 25-hour day, zeitgebers pull you back into the standard 24-hour day.

Among the strongest zeitgebers, sleep scientists have found, is very bright light, either sunlight or light up to 200 times brighter than normal indoor light. Such light is often used to "reset" circadian rhythms run amok, as with delayed sleep phase syndrome (DSPS) in which you can't fall asleep until later than you'd like to. For more on this condition, see page 156.

Juggling Jet Lag

Jet lag is a perfect example of circadian rhythms gone haywire. You know you've had it if you've ever flown from New York to London and spent half your weeklong vacation "recovering" from the travel hangover, only to have it hit again once you're home. When you pass from one time zone to another, your circadian rhythms get out of tune. Traveling from California to New York, for example, causes you to "lose" three hours according to your body's clock. You'll feel tired when the alarm rings at 8:00 the next morning because, according to your body's clock, it's still 5:00. It usually takes several days for your cycles to adjust to the new time. It's generally easier to travel from east to west—because you're pushing your body clock ahead instead of back. The most common effects of jet lag include fatigue, sleep disturbances, insomnia, mild depression, irritability, gastrointestinal distress, and headaches.

To reduce the effects of jet lag, some doctors try to manipulate the biological clock with light therapy, exposing people to special lights many times brighter than ordinary household light for several hours near the time the subjects want to wake up. This helps them reset their biological clocks and adjust to a new time zone. Left to your own devices, it generally takes one day to adjust for every time zone you crossed.

There are several things you can do for yourself to counteract the effects of jet lag:

Pay off your sleep debt. Your jet lag will be worse if you're tired before you leave for your trip.

Adjust your preflight sleep schedule. If you're traveling westward, for instance, try going to bed 15 minutes later and getting up 15 minutes later (adding another 15 minutes each day) every day for a week.

Stick to your home schedule. For short trips, some travelers remain on their home schedule, sleeping when they'd normally sleep at home, even if it's still daylight at their destination. This may be difficult to do, however, if you have meetings or other time-sensitive commitments.

Adopt the new schedule. Adopt the schedule of your destination as quickly as possible. If your New York body clock says it's 10 p.m., but your London clock says it's 5 p.m., plan dinner, not bedtime.

Get some sun. Sunlight, as discussed earlier, is a zeitgeber that helps reset your body clock. If you arrive at your destination during daylight hours, get out and take a walk. Exposure to bright light in the morning helps you shift forward, so you can go to bed later and wake up earlier. Bright light in the evening shifts you back, so you can go to sleep earlier and wake up later.

Work out. Exercise helps reset your circadian rhythms and will also keep you awake until your new bedtime

Eat lightly. It is important to eat lightly at the beginning of your trip. Your stomach may not be able to handle heavy meals until your body clock is reset.

Nap. Try just a brief nap upon arrival, especially if you're flying eastward. This can give you just enough sleep reserve to make it through until bedtime in your destination. Some hotels even offer "jet lag" rooms with special blackout curtains and full-spectrum light, as well as 24-hour room service (so you can have "dinner" at 7 a.m.).

Shifting Rhythms Due to Shift Work

In the arena of circadian rhythm disrupters, shift work—when you work nights and sleep days—wins top awards, literally turning your circadian rhythms on their head. Yet the whole phenomenon of shift work is relatively new. As Dr. Dement notes in *The Promise of Sleep*, before World War II few people worked at night. With the advent of the war economy and 24-hour factories, everything changed. Today, Bureau of Labor statistics show an estimated 17 percent of employees work swing shifts (typically from 4 p.m. to midnight) or night shifts (generally from midnight to 8 a.m.).

What's worse, many people are forced to switch shifts on a regular basis, which causes their circadian rhythms to go haywire.

As Dr. Dement notes, changing shifts is like flying through eight time zones, the equivalent of flying from Denver to Tokyo or from San Francisco to London. It's no surprise that shift workers tend to experience symptoms similar to jet lag. Because their work schedules are at odds with powerful sleep-regulating cues like sunlight, they often become tired during work and suffer insomnia or other problems when trying to sleep. They also have an increased risk of heart problems, digestive disturbances, and emotional and mental problems, all of which may be related to their sleeping problems. The number and severity of workplace accidents tends to increase during the night shift. Major industrial accidents attributed in part to errors made by fatigued night-shift workers include the *Exxon Valdez* oil spill and the Three Mile Island and Chernobyl nuclear power plant accidents. One study also found that medical interns working on the night shift are twice as likely as others to misinterpret hospital test records, which could endanger their patients.

In addition to problems with circadian rhythms, shift workers must also cope with the difficulties inherent in trying to sleep when the rest of the world is awake. As night owl Donna, described earlier in this chapter, notes, "Don't let anybody tell you suburbia is a quiet place, at least not during the day. Neighbors are mowing lawns, UPS guys are delivering packages, and somebody is always calling—invariably in the morning. And then there's the light. I thought we'd get used to it, but even after two years, we find it tough to get to a very deep state of sleep when it's light an hour or two after we get to bed. While we've made getting enough sleep a priority in our lives, because of all we have to do and all the interruptions, we still often feel jet-lagged, and one or the other of us sometimes has insomnia."

Several consultant organizations, including Circadian Technologies, Inc., have sprung up to counsel organizations on how to handle their shift workers in an effort to reduce turnover and accidents while improving productivity. Circadian recommends employers do the following:

- Conduct mandated training on the night shift rather than requiring employees to upset their routine and train on the day shift.
- Add a fitness room with treadmill, recumbent bicycle, and weight-training equipment.
- Install natural-light bulbs in continuously occupied areas.
- Improve overhead lighting.
- Provide counseling and training in lieu of discipline for minor or isolated errors.
- Provide hot chocolate along with coffee and tea.
- Set up a stereo in the control room.
- Change shift changeover time on a 12-hour schedule from midnight and noon to 6 a.m. and 6 p.m.
- Encourage employees to do more strenuous work early in the 12-hour shift.
- Change from a backward rotating schedule (days to nights to evenings) to a forward rotation (days to evenings to nights).

The Stages of Sleep

While your internal clock determines your sleep schedule, electrical changes in your brain determine the quality of your sleep as you gradually move back and forth between five different sleep phases: stages 1 through 4 and REM (rapid eye movement) sleep, when the most vivid dreams occur. They progress in a cycle from stage 1 to REM sleep, then start over again with stage 1. We spend almost half our total sleep time in stage 2, about 20 to 25 percent in REM sleep, and the remainder in the other stages. A complete cycle takes an average of 90 to 110 minutes.

The first sleep cycles each night contain relatively short REM periods and long periods of deep sleep (stages 3 and 4). As the night progresses, REM sleep periods increase in length while deep sleep decreases. By morning, you're spending nearly all your sleep time in stages 1, 2, and REM, which may be why you can often remember your dreams when you wake up in the morning.

Here's how it breaks down:

Stage 1. This is light sleep, or dozing. You're drifting in and out of sleep and can be awakened easily. Your eyes move very slowly and your muscle activity slows. If you're awakened from stage 1 sleep, you may remember fragmented visual images. Some people also have sudden muscle contractions similar to the way you'd react if startled, called hypnic myoclonia, often preceded by a sensation of starting to fall.

Stage 2. In this stage, your eye movements stop and your brain waves become slower, with occasional bursts of electrical activity called sleep spindles. This marks the beginning of real sleep.

Stage 3. In this stage, extremely slow brain waves called delta waves (very low-frequency, high-voltage) begin to appear, interspersed with smaller, faster waves.

Stage 4. By this stage, your brain produces delta waves almost exclusively. It is very difficult to wake someone during stages 3 and 4, when one is in a state of deep sleep. There is no eye movement or muscle activity. If you wake up during these stages you'll feel groggy and disoriented for several minutes. This is when children experience bedwetting, night terrors, or sleep walking. This is the restorative phase of sleep, when the body repairs itself. If this stage of sleep is disturbed, even if you spend eight hours sleeping, you'll still feel tired the next day.

REM sleep. When you switch into REM sleep, your breathing becomes more rapid, irregular, and shallow. Your eyes jerk rapidly in various directions, and your limb muscles become temporarily paralyzed. Your heart rate increases, your blood pressure rises, and men have erections. When people are awakened during REM sleep, they often describe bizarre and illogical tales or dreams. The first REM sleep usually occurs about 70 to 90 minutes after you fall asleep. If your REM sleep is disrupted one night, your body doesn't follow the normal sleep cycle progression the next time you doze off. Instead, you often slip directly into REM sleep and go through extended periods of REM until you "catch up" on this stage of sleep.

REM sleep stimulates the brain regions used in learning. This may be important for normal brain development during infancy, which would explain why infants spend much more time in REM sleep than adults. One study found that REM sleep affects how you learn certain mental skills. People taught a skill and then deprived of non-REM sleep could recall what they had learned after sleeping, while people deprived of REM sleep could not.

People who are under anesthesia or in a coma are often said to be asleep. However, they cannot be awakened and don't produce the complex, active brain wave patterns seen in normal sleep. Instead, their brain waves are very slow and weak, sometimes barely detectable.

Dreaming the Night Away

We typically spend more than two hours each night dreaming, yet very little is known about how or why we dream. Sigmund Freud believed dreaming was a "safety valve" for unconscious desires. Only after 1953, when researchers first described REM in sleeping infants, did scientists begin to study sleep and dreaming. They soon realized that the strange, illogical experiences we call dreams almost always occur during REM sleep. While most mammals and birds show signs of REM sleep, reptiles and other cold-blooded animals don't.

Dr. Dement, one of the first to discover that even newborn babies dream, calls dreaming "a form of awareness, an ability to put together sensory information and thoughts in a way that mimics what happens when we are awake."

REM sleep begins with signals from an area at the base of the brain called the pons. These signals travel to a brain region called the thalamus, which relays them to the cerebral cortex—the outer layer of the brain responsible for learning, thinking, and organizing information. The pons also sends signals that shut off neurons in the spinal cord, causing temporary paralysis of the limb muscles. If something interferes with this paralysis, people begin to physically "act out" their dreams—a rare, dangerous problem called REM sleep behavior disorder. A person dreaming about a ball game, for example, may run headlong into furniture or blindly strike someone sleeping nearby while trying to catch a ball in the dream.

Some scientists believe dreams are the cortex's attempt to find meaning in the random signals that it receives during REM sleep. The cortex is the part of the brain that interprets and organizes information from the environment during consciousness. It may be that, given random signals from the pons during REM sleep, the cortex tries to interpret these signals as well, creating a "story" out of fragmented brain activity.

Sleep Needs Change As We Age

As anyone who has ever had a child knows, our sleep needs change as we age. Infants, for instance, spend between 16 and 18 hours a day sleeping, divided into six or seven sessions, with nearly half their time asleep spent in REM sleep. Compare that to the seven hours of sleep most middle-aged adults get, with just 20 to 25 percent spent in REM, or the 15 to 20 percent older adults spend in REM sleep.

By the end of the first year, babies are still sleeping about 16 hours a day, but it tends to be more organized sleep, with a morning and afternoon nap breaking up periods of wakefulness. By the end of their second year, most children have given up the morning nap, and sleep about 12 hours. By age four or five, the afternoon nap is also gone, and children are sleeping about ten hours a night. This remains steady until children reach puberty. Dr. Dement calls the sleep of childhood the "Golden Age" of sleep, when most of the sleep problems that plague adults are nonexistent. Children play and work hard all day, full of energy, then fall asleep almost immediately, sleeping soundly throughout the night.

When the roller coaster of adolescence begins, teenagers shift into an entirely different sleep pattern as their bodies release a flood of hormones during sleep to get them through puberty. So much of growth and development depends on sleep during this phase that, for teens, not getting enough sleep can actually stunt growth. In recent years, several studies on adolescent sleep patterns revealed that teenagers need as much sleep as younger children, but rarely get it, and so carry tremendous levels of sleep debt, which interferes with their ability to learn. This sleep debt increases the likelihood that teenagers will become aggressive or violent and develop sleep disorders. In one study, students who described themselves as struggling or failing in school (Cs, Ds, Fs) reported that they slept about 25 minutes less, and went to bed an average of 40 minutes later on school nights than students getting As and Bs.

Studies on adolescents also found that teenagers have a different sleep clock than younger children or adults; they tend to get a burst of energy in the early evening, feeling wide awake into the late evening when most of us are very sleepy, and thus need to sleep later in the morning. At least one school district in Minnesota has changed the starting time for its high school students from 7:20 to 8:30 a.m. as a result of this research. Today school officials report that students are more awake and behavioral problems have decreased, notes Dr. Dement.

Once we move through adolescence, though, we tend to sleep less. The older we get, it seems the less we sleep overall. This is due not so much to lifestyle, but to changes in circadian rhythms. Older adults begin going to bed earlier and sleeping less. Even very healthy older people, researchers report, spend about 90 minutes or more of the night awake and often make up for the lack of sleep with daytime naps.

Making Good Use of Naps

I have a confession to make. My idea of indulgence is not a bubble bath or a massage; it's a nap. And one of the best things about being a writer and working from home is that I can take a nap every day. On the couch in the den, under my fuzzy mohair blanket, my snoring dog at my feet. I wake from that hour in the dark (often spending just 20 minutes of it asleep) as refreshed as if I've had a full night's sleep. If I miss my daily nap, I'm a mess for the rest of the afternoon and evening, often with a horrible headache and a chronic inability to focus or restrain my crankiness.

According to the research, I'm not alone. Large-scale surveys find that about 90 percent of all adults experience sleepiness after lunch. But it's not the lunch that makes us sleepy; it's our sleep debt coupled with a natural tendency for our circadian rhythms to dip in early afternoon.

Some athletes, like former professional mountain biker and Olympian Ruthe Matthes, take midday naps as a routine part of their training to give their bodies time to restore and heal. In fact, New England Patriots' quarterback Tom Brady, who led his team to victory in the 2002 Super Bowl, said he napped in the locker room before the game and "woke up calm and confident." President George W. Bush has said that, in addition to his reported 10 p.m. bedtime, he regularly takes afternoon power naps.

Thankfully, more employers are recognizing that a brief nap can provide benefits in terms of more productive employees. My own former employer had an actual nap room, with a comfortable couch, blanket, and blackout blinds.

All stages of sleep are important, but the sleep that helps your body recover happens quite soon after falling asleep. That's

> why naps pack so much power—because those first 20 to 30 minutes of sleep are so critical. The best time to take a nap is from noon to 6 p.m., with the peak time from 1 to 3 p.m. The ideal nap is just 20 minutes long, so you don't move into the deep sleep phases.

What About Sleep Medication?

"My sleep-deprived or should I say 'sleep-depraved' daughter, tried Tylenol PM. She missed classes the other morning because she took two and slept through two alarms!"
—Mary Jo Schulze, Nazareth, Pa.

"I have no idea if this is a proven remedy everyone else in the world knows about, or even if it works for anyone else. And I have no idea if a doctor would say it is safe or silly . . . but, I've found that if I'm all wired before my regular bedtime, if I take two plain-ole Bayer Aspirin, in about fifteen minutes I get very, very sleepy. I figure it is much safer than a real sleeping pill."
—Veda Eddy, Iowa City

How many times have you reached for a pill when you had trouble falling asleep? From over-the-counter medications like Tylenol PM and Sominex, to the newer prescription sleep medications like Sonata (zaleplon), better sleep through chemicals seems to be an option of choice for millions of insomnia-plagued Americans. One-fifth of adults (22 percent) say they've taken medication to help them sleep, according to the National Sleep Foundation's 2000 "Sleep in America" omnibus poll. In 1995, Americans spent $1.97 billion on the pharmacologic treatment of insomnia.

Of those who did use a medication to help them sleep, most used over-the-counter medications (56 percent), including herbal medications (more on these on Day 3 of the Seven-Day Sleep Program), and about one-third used prescription medications. A few (10 percent) used both. One reason few adults say they'd use a sleeping pill if they can't sleep is their concern that, if they start using sleeping pills, they might always need them to sleep.

There's nothing wrong with occasionally turning to a pill when you're suffering from intermittent insomnia. Sometimes, the good night's sleep it may provide is all you need to break the pattern of insomnia. However, it becomes a problem if you're turning to supplements and medications for chronic insomnia, or every time you have problem sleeping. Then sleeping medications can, themselves, become the cause of the insomnia. Continue taking the medications, particularly prescription medications, and your body builds up a tolerance, requiring you to take increasing doses. When you finally try to stop taking them, the insomnia returns with a vengeance in a situation called "rebound" insomnia, or "drug dependency insomnia." Some studies found just three days of sleeping medications can result in this rebound effect.

The Seven-Day Sleep Program is designed to provide you with a long-term, natural approach to a good night's sleep. However, no sleep book would be complete without some explanation of the myriad of prescription and over-the-counter sleep aids currently available. Ideally, once you finish the program, you can trash all your pills!

Over-the-Counter Medications

There are a variety of over-the-counter medications, ranging from Tylenol PM to Sominex and Nytol, that claim to induce sleep. All work the same way: They contain an antihistamine. That's why over-the-counter antihistamines taken for allergies, like Benadryl, make you so sleepy. In fact, I've used Benadryl as a sleep aid for my children when they were young and we had a long plane ride ahead. One child-sized dose and they slept like, well, babies, throughout the flight. Most pharmacists and doctors, however, say these medications don't work well as sleep aids for adults. You can build up a tolerance to them, and side effects include constipation, dry mouth, anxiety, and possible "rebound" insomnia once you stop taking them.

Prescription Medications

Your doctor has a plethora of anxiety-reducing and sleep-enhancing prescriptions he or she can prescribe. Only you and your doctor know what's right for you. Among the options are:

Antianxiety drugs or sedatives (benzodiazepines). These medications work on certain neurotransmitters within the brain called GABA to relax and soothe you, often all you need in order to fall asleep. However, some can be highly addictive, leaving you with a "hangover" in the morning. They are used only for a short time—about two weeks on average—and should only be used for short-term insomnia. These drugs include Xanax (alprazolam), Valium (diazepam), Ativan (lorazepam), and BuSpar (buspirone).

Sleeping pills. Contrary to popular belief, today's sleeping pills are not addicting. Still, when Dr. Dement surveyed students in one of his classes at Stanford University, 94 percent agreed with the statement "sleeping pills are addictive," and three-fourths agreed with the statement, "Sleeping pills should not be taken unless you have had difficulty sleeping for more than a month." Neither of these statements is correct.

A study of 500 primary-care physicians around the country found that 90 percent also believed that sleep medications are addicting and have serious side effects. As Dr. Dement notes in *The Promise of Sleep*, at a government hearing about the use of Halcion as a sleep aid, one doctor said, "Using a sleeping pill is like swatting a mosquito with a sledgehammer." This misconception could prevent you from receiving a much-needed prescription for your transient insomnia.

In general, these drugs are prescribed at the lowest dose and for the shortest duration needed to relieve the sleep-related symptoms. With some, the dose must be lowered gradually as the medicine is discontinued because, if stopped abruptly, it can cause insomnia to occur again for a night or two. When considering a prescription sleep aid, one of the most important things to know is how long the active ingredient remains active in your body. That will determine how well you function the next day.

Ideally, the type of sleeping pill your doctor prescribes should depend on your particular sleep problem, says Joyce A. Walsleben, author of *A Woman's Guide to Sleep*. "Remember that while using any sleeping pill, you may have episodes of amnesia or poor coordination if you awaken and try to function," she warns. "So choose your nights wisely, and don't take sleep medication on a night during which you may be awakened, or are alone with young children."

Dr. Walsleben divides prescription sleeping medications into the following categories:

For problems falling asleep. Short-acting sedatives like Halcion (triaxolam), Ambien (zolpidem), or Sonata (zaleplon) work for up to four hours. The newest drug, Sonata, apparently has few-to-no lingering effects, with those taking it in clinical trials functioning normally even when they're awakened one hour after taking it.

For problems staying asleep. Longer-acting drugs like Restoril (temazepam) or Dalmane (flurazepam) may help. These are sedating benzodiazepines, which may be still working when you get up in the morning, leading to the sleeping pill "hangover." Another option is to simply take another dose of the short-acting medication Sonata when you're wakeful, suggests Dr. Walsleben.

Other medications. Some antidepressants can aid sleep, generally with minimal side effects. They're particularly helpful if you're suffering from depression, which often disrupts sleep. Some of the sedating antidepressants include Remeron (mirtazapine), Desyrel (trazodone), and Serzone (nefazodone).

BENZODIAZEPINES USED IN THE TREATMENT OF INSOMNIA

Medication	Dosage	Peak action	Half-life*
Estazolam (Prosom)	1 to 2 mg	2 hours	10 to 24 hours
Flurazepam (Dalmane)	15 to 30 mg	0.5 to 1 hour	2 to 3 hours
Oxazepam (Serax)	10 to 15 mg	3 hours	5 to 10 hours
Quazepam (Doral)	7.5 to 15 mg	2 hours	41 hours
Temazepam (Restoril)	7.5 mg to 30 mg	1.2 to 1.6 hours	3.5 to 18.4 hours
Triazolam (Halcion)	0.125 to 0.5 mg	1 to 2 hours	1.5 to 5.5 hours
Zolpidem (Ambien)	5 to 10 mg	1.6 hours	2.5 hours

Source: American Family Physician

*The time required for half the amount of medication to be eliminated from your body.

To help you track your own sleep habits, the next chapter describes how to maintain a sleep log, or diary. Your diary will provide invaluable information as you work your way through the Seven-Day Sleep Program.

Three

Getting Started on Your Sleep Diary

"After years of believing I needed eight hours of sleep every night, I finally discovered that I feel far more rested and energetic when I cut that down to six and a half or seven. Feeling more rested on less sleep—what could be better?"
—Miranda, 48

"If I don't get at least eight hours, I simply cannot function."
—Marsha Shapiro, Atlanta

SO YOU WOKE UP THIS MORNING CONVINCED YOU'D tossed and turned all night, but your partner insists you snored right through the baby's screams. Or, for the past two weeks, you've suddenly had trouble falling asleep, yet you can't think of anything in your life that's different. That's where a sleep diary comes in.

In this chapter, you'll learn how a sleep diary can help you understand your own sleep problems and pinpoint the sleep issues you need to address through the Seven-Day Sleep Program. You'll get a sample sleep diary, and detailed instructions on how to complete it.

How Much Sleep Do You Need?

How much sleep adults need is the subject of great debate, particularly since the publication of a highly controversial study in early 2002 that found those who got more than eight hours of sleep a night were likely to die sooner than those who had less sleep. Don't worry, the study itself was flawed. But it did raise the difficult-to-answer question about how much sleep the average adult needs. The answer, it seems, is as individual as the sleeper. Overall, sleep experts agree that most healthy adults need about eight hours of sleep a night, although research finds actual amounts for individuals range from four to ten hours a night.

So how do you know how much sleep you really need? Next time you're on vacation, note when you go to bed, then allow yourself to sleep as long as you want in the morning. By the end of the week, when you've lowered your sleep debt, you should be sleeping the number of hours just right for you. Of course, this only works if you're not an insomniac.

If you don't have a vacation coming up, begin monitoring your sleep at home, tracking it in the sleep diary provided below. Go to bed eight hours before you have to wake up. Do this for several nights in a row, and observe how tired you feel throughout the day. If you're still feeling sleepy by the evening, try going to bed a half hour earlier, then a half hour earlier the next night, and so on until you reach the point at which you feel well rested the following day. Conversely, if you go to bed expecting eight hours of sleep, and lie awake for 45 minutes, consider cutting down the time you spend in bed until you find that perfect equilibrium.

Sleep experts refer to "sleep architecture," which covers how long it takes you to fall asleep, how much time you spend in each sleep stage (see Chapter 2), how many times you wake up at night, and how long you remain awake. All play a role in your overall sleep quality and any resulting sleep debt. One goal of the Seven-Day Sleep Program is to strengthen the foundation of your sleep architecture to help reduce your sleep debt.

Tracking Your Sleep: The Sleep Diary

Some might call Kate Bramson, 31, a bit obsessive about her sleep habits. Kate began tracking her sleep patterns while on the high school fencing team. She was curious to see whether she followed a more regimented schedule, and therefore got more sleep, when she was busier. While she never added up the hours to see if she really did get more sleep when she was on the team, she found she liked keeping track of her sleep habits, being able to look back and see that on a particular day she went to bed earlier than she had in months. "It was just fun to keep track," she says, "and it became a habit."

At first she tracked her sleep on Post-it-sized notepaper, cramming as many weeks as she could onto each piece of paper. Today, she jots down notes on a pocket calendar, tracking when she goes to sleep and wakes up, including any middle-of-the-night awakenings, circling the total amount of sleep she gets each day. Flipping through the year 2000, for instance, she can see that her sleep ranged from 14 or even 15 hours a day when she was diagnosed with mononucleosis in January to a more typical eight hours once she recovered.

The diary enabled her to see that at her sickest, she was sleeping 70 hours a week, and that once she started feeling better, she settled into a pattern of about 58 hours a week, which she's decided is best for her. "Consequently, if I notice that there's a week where I only get 50 hours of sleep, I try to make that up in the next week by sleeping more than 65 hours," she says.

Between January and February 2001, shortly after she and her husband bought and began restoring their first house, she realized she was about 30 hours in sleep debt. "I embarked on an effort to make up my sleep debt and tried to go to bed each night at 9 p.m. and get up at 7 a.m.," she said. "For the first week, I slept 70 hours and felt much better." Unfortunately, the following week the 2002 Winter Olympics began, and her carefully constructed sleep plan was shattered.

Kate uses her sleep diary much as sleep researchers do—to track sleep patterns that might point to a problem. In fact, if you go to see a sleep specialist about your sleeping problems, the first thing you'll be asked to do is keep a sleep diary, or log. And that's just what we want you to do here, before you start the Seven-Day Sleep Program.

Keeping Your Sleep Diary

"A sleep diary is like looking in the mirror at your sleep habits," says Michael D. Weinstein, M.D., director of the division of pulmonary and critical care medicine at Winthrop University Hospital's Sleep Disorders Center in Mineola, New York. "The diary should include simple things, like what time you go to bed, how long it takes you to fall asleep, how many times you awaken during the night, and how long you're awake when you do wake up."

Dr. Weinstein cautions against becoming too focused on the details or the diary. "Many patients who complain of insomnia are overly fixated on their sleep anyway," he says. "Their life revolves around this difficulty. You don't want to get them even more fixated on chronicling every detail. So we're looking for more of a ballpark feeling, like did you wake up once or six times, how long do you estimate you stayed awake, etc."

It's also important to note what you do when you wake up in the middle of the night Dr. Weinstein says. Do you just lie there, dozing on and off? Do you watch TV, read, get out of bed, or have a snack? Just as important are details about your physical environment: Is it too hot or cold or noisy? Is your partner snoring or restless?

Also keep track of:

- What, how much, and when you last ate and drank, what you ate during the day. List all caffeinated beverages and foods, including coffee, tea, and soft drinks.
- What medications you took. Include aspirin and other over-the-counter medications which could contain caffeine, as well as all prescription medications, vitamins, and other supplements.
- How many cigarettes you smoked during the day. What time you smoked your last cigarette.
- Whom you sleep with, including pets. Does your sleeping partner (or pet) snore, roll over a lot, or suffer from insomnia?
- How you feel when you wake up: refreshed, tired?
- How much and what type of exercise you do during the day, as well as the time of exercise.
- Nap times and duration.

It's important that you fill in your sleep diary every morning as soon as you wake up, with your night fresh in your mind, and every evening before going to bed, while your day is still fresh in your mind. If you awaken in the middle of the night, try to jot down the time. Make a note of how long you were awake, if you can, before falling asleep again.

Track how you feel throughout the day. If you're excessively sleepy, it's a clear sign that your sleep the night before wasn't sufficient, which may indicate a medical problem, particularly if you think you slept long enough.

Your diary may show that you couldn't lie still, a possible sign of restless legs syndrome, described in more detail in Chapter 5. Or it may indicate that you're getting up to drink large amounts of water at night, a possible sign of diabetes.

Try to vary your patterns. If you never exercise, try exercising two or three days while you're keeping the log so you can see if it makes a difference in your sleep. If you drink a Diet Coke every night with dinner, followed by a cup of coffee, cut them out for a couple of nights to see if it makes a difference in your sleep.

After you've completed a week's worth of logs, sit down with a highlighter and go through each day looking for patterns. If you slept well on Tuesday but poorly on Wednesday, what was different about the two days? Did you exercise, have an unusually stressful day at work, a fight with your teenager or spouse? Highlight the differences, and see if patterns appear.

Don't stop keeping your diary once you start the Seven-Day Sleep Program. This is where the diary becomes even more important. It will clearly show you what works and what doesn't in terms of improving your sleep. Even people who swear that the lifestyle changes they make aren't working are surprised to see they're sleeping more soundly, or getting more sleep, when they look back at their diaries.

Here is a sample sleep diary. Make several copies of this diary and track your sleep habits for at least a week. That should be enough time to highlight any patterns of behavior or environmental issues that are causing you problems with sleeping.

COMPLETE IN MORNING

	I went to bed last night at:	I got out of bed this morning at:	Last night I fell asleep in:	I woke up during the night: (Record number of times)	When I woke up for the day, I felt: (Check one)	Last night I slept for a total of: (Record number of hours)	My sleep was disturbed by: (List any mental, emotional, physical, or enviromental factores that affected your sleep, e.g. stress, snoring, physical discomfort, temperature)
Day 1 DAY _____ DATE _____	PM / AM	AM / PM	MINUTES	TIMES	___ REFRESHED ___ SOMEWHAT REFRESHED ___ FATIGUED	HOURS	
Day 2 DAY _____ DATE _____	PM / AM	AM / PM	MINUTES	TIMES	___ REFRESHED ___ SOMEWHAT REFRESHED ___ FATIGUED	HOURS	
Day 3 DAY _____ DATE _____	PM / AM	AM / PM	MINUTES	TIMES	___ REFRESHED ___ SOMEWHAT REFRESHED ___ FATIGUED	HOURS	
Day 4 DAY _____ DATE _____	PM / AM	AM / PM	MINUTES	TIMES	___ REFRESHED ___ SOMEWHAT REFRESHED ___ FATIGUED	HOURS	
Day 5 DAY _____ DATE _____	PM / AM	AM / PM	MINUTES	TIMES	___ REFRESHED ___ SOMEWHAT REFRESHED ___ FATIGUED	HOURS	
Day 6 DAY _____ DATE _____	PM / AM	AM / PM	MINUTES	TIMES	___ REFRESHED ___ SOMEWHAT REFRESHED ___ FATIGUED	HOURS	
Day 7 DAY _____ DATE _____	PM / AM	AM / PM	MINUTES	TIMES	___ REFRESHED ___ SOMEWHAT REFRESHED ___ FATIGUED	HOURS	

COMPLETE AT THE END OF DAY

	I consumed caffeinated drinks in the:	I exercised at least 20 minutes in the:	Approximately 2-3 hours before going to bed, I consumed:	Medication(s) I took during the day: [List name of medication/drug(s)]	About 1 hour before going to sleep, I did the following activity: (List activity, e.g. watch TV, work, read)
Day 1 DAY _____ DATE _____	__ MORNING __ AFTERNOON __ 2-3 HOURS BEFORE GOING TO BED __ NOT APPLICABLE	__ MORNING __ AFTERNOON __ 2-3 HOURS BEFORE GOING TO BED __ NOT APPLICABLE	__ ALCOHOL __ A HEAVY MEAL __ NOT APPLICABLE	_____ _____ _____ _____	_____ _____ _____ _____
Day 2 DAY _____ DATE _____	__ MORNING __ AFTERNOON __ 2-3 HOURS BEFORE GOING TO BED __ NOT APPLICABLE	__ MORNING __ AFTERNOON __ 2-3 HOURS BEFORE GOING TO BED __ NOT APPLICABLE	__ ALCOHOL __ A HEAVY MEAL __ NOT APPLICABLE	_____ _____ _____ _____	_____ _____ _____ _____
Day 3 DAY _____ DATE _____	__ MORNING __ AFTERNOON __ 2-3 HOURS BEFORE GOING TO BED __ NOT APPLICABLE	__ MORNING __ AFTERNOON __ 2-3 HOURS BEFORE GOING TO BED __ NOT APPLICABLE	__ ALCOHOL __ A HEAVY MEAL __ NOT APPLICABLE	_____ _____ _____ _____	_____ _____ _____ _____
Day 4 DAY _____ DATE _____	__ MORNING __ AFTERNOON __ 2-3 HOURS BEFORE GOING TO BED __ NOT APPLICABLE	__ MORNING __ AFTERNOON __ 2-3 HOURS BEFORE GOING TO BED __ NOT APPLICABLE	__ ALCOHOL __ A HEAVY MEAL __ NOT APPLICABLE	_____ _____ _____ _____	_____ _____ _____ _____
Day 5 DAY _____ DATE _____	__ MORNING __ AFTERNOON __ 2-3 HOURS BEFORE GOING TO BED __ NOT APPLICABLE	__ MORNING __ AFTERNOON __ 2-3 HOURS BEFORE GOING TO BED __ NOT APPLICABLE	__ ALCOHOL __ A HEAVY MEAL __ NOT APPLICABLE	_____ _____ _____ _____	_____ _____ _____ _____
Day 6 DAY _____ DATE _____	__ MORNING __ AFTERNOON __ 2-3 HOURS BEFORE GOING TO BED __ NOT APPLICABLE	__ MORNING __ AFTERNOON __ 2-3 HOURS BEFORE GOING TO BED __ NOT APPLICABLE	__ ALCOHOL __ A HEAVY MEAL __ NOT APPLICABLE	_____ _____ _____ _____	_____ _____ _____ _____
Day 7 DAY _____ DATE _____	__ MORNING __ AFTERNOON __ 2-3 HOURS BEFORE GOING TO BED __ NOT APPLICABLE	__ MORNING __ AFTERNOON __ 2-3 HOURS BEFORE GOING TO BED __ NOT APPLICABLE	__ ALCOHOL __ A HEAVY MEAL __ NOT APPLICABLE	_____ _____ _____ _____	_____ _____ _____ _____

Before You Start the Seven-Day Sleep Program: Get a Tune Up

Once your diary is complete, and before you start the Seven-Day Sleep Program, it's a good idea to consult your physician to make sure you don't have a physical, treatable problem that can be corrected with medication, surgery, or other medical options. Once you've taken that step—and completed your diary—you're ready to begin the program.

Four

The Seven-Day Sleep Program

DAY 1: SETTING THE STAGE FOR A GOOD NIGHT'S SLEEP

TODAY, ON THE FIRST DAY OF THE SEVEN-DAY SLEEP program, you're going to evaluate your bedroom from top to bottom, making some simple changes to prepare for tonight's sleep. Then you'll make a list of future changes to implement during the coming weeks.

For some reason, the bedroom seems to be the last room most people furnish. They'll spend thousands getting the kitchen, family room, and bathrooms just perfect, while still sleeping on the hand-me-down mattress their in-laws donated when they got married. Yet, as noted earlier, we easily spend one-third of our lives in the bedroom—more time than in any other room of the house. So why don't we spend the money and make the effort to ensure that every element of the room—from the decor to the furniture to the lighting—is designed to enhance its primary purpose? Especially since, as one survey found, at least one out of four people say their sleep is frequently sabotaged by environmental factors in the bedroom—whether it's light, noise, temperature, or an uncomfortable mattress.

Only after suffering through countless sleepless mornings did night owls Donna and Ray, the couple we met in Chapter 2 who sleep much of the morning and are awake most of the night, rearrange their bedroom to enhance their daytime sleep. "We put the bed on an adjacent wall to prevent the sun's shining in our eyes in the morning, and equipped the bedroom with a humidifier to make the room feel more comfortable," Donna said. "Believe it or not, we both feel we've slept better since we bought it. We're also in the process of buying floor-length blackout curtains (which fit under regular curtains) for our bedroom."

With her changes, Donna is addressing the three environmental toxins that most interfere with sleep: noise, light, and temperature. But there are other aspects of your bedroom—from the kind of pillow you use to the brightness of the glow-in-the-dark numerals of your alarm clock—that can interfere with a good night's sleep.

Review and Reflect

Now you'll see the benefits of keeping that sleep diary. Turn to your diary, and look for any indication that your sleep environment plays havoc with your rest. Did you note that you had trouble getting comfortable? Maybe you need a new mattress. Did you wake up one night because you were too hot? Grab an extra blanket because the temperature dropped? When you woke up in the middle of the night, did you find your eyes drawn to the glowing red numbers on your bedside clock, the flashing clock on the VCR, or the hulking shape of your computer reminding you of work undone? Even if you simply noted that you woke up an hour before your alarm went off because the sun was in your eyes, this is an important clue to changes you need to make in your sleep environment.

Be flexible with the advice given on this first day. The best environment for your best night's sleep is the one that works for you. Who knows, maybe the sounds of silence really are too noisy for you.

Evaluate Your Bedroom

The checklist below will help you identify problem areas in your bedroom. Make a copy of this list (or use the one right out of the book) and, starting in one corner of your bedroom, work your way around the room evaluating every aspect.

Answer each question as honestly and fully as possible.

My bedroom contains:
> A television and VCR/DVD
> A computer
> My work desk

My windows are covered by:
> Nothing
> A sheet
> Sheer curtains
> Heavy drapes
> Blinds
> Shades
> Blackout curtains

My mattress is:
> 1–5 years old
> 6–10 years old
> Older than my teenager

I turn my mattress:
> Every month
> Every six months

Every year
You're supposed to turn your mattress?
My bedroom is painted _____.
When I lie in bed at night, I hear _____.
When I walk into my bedroom I smell _____.
When I walk into my bedroom I feel _____.
My bedroom temperature is always:
  Hot
  Cold
  Just right
The bed in my bedroom faces _____.

Once you've completed your checklist, you're ready for the next steps.

Consider Your Mattress

> *"The biggest thing I've done to promote a good night's sleep is get a new mattress. Our new mattress has improved our sleep and it feels so wonderful that we now refer to our bed as bed-opia."*
> —Vicky Mlyniec, Los Gatos, Calif.

A survey of 400 adults conducted by ARC Consulting for the Better Sleep Council found that eight in ten believed sleep problems could be caused by a poor mattress, and nearly half described the condition of their current mattress as "bad" or "very bad" when they finally bought a new one.

You need a new mattress (and the box spring that goes with it) if:

- Your mattress is ten years old or more;
- It has formed peaks, valleys, or lumps, or has other visible signs of wear and tear;
- You wake up feeling stiff, sore, or achy.

Before you shop, determine what size mattress you need. As you'll learn in Day 6 of the Seven-Day Sleep Program, sleeping with someone can significantly disturb your sleep. So make sure you get a mattress that's large enough. One study found that the longer you live with someone, the bigger the bed you eventually wind up with. Overall, 49 percent of couples sleep on a queen-size mattress, and 31 percent on a king-size. If you're planning to stick with your full-sized mattress, consider this: You and your partner each have only as much room to move around in as a baby has in a crib.

Once you've determined what size mattress you want, you next need to consider what type of mattress is best. Among the key considerations:

Support. Firm or soft? Pillow-top or flat? You want a mattress that gently supports your body at all points and keeps your spine in the same position as a good standing posture. The few valid studies of mattresses have failed to show that the type or the firmness influences sleep, although a softer mattress may limit your natural nighttime movement, making it hard to get comfortable.

When *Consumer Reports* tested mattresses, it found that a firmer mattress won't resist permanent body sagging better than a softer mattress; that a thicker mattress sags more than a thinner one; and that because all the permanent compression is within the padding layers, not the springs, more padding equals more potential for sagging. So go with whatever feels good to you. It is a good idea to try out the mattress in the store, something customers are surprisingly loath to do. We spend more time test driving a car than we do a mattress, yet we spend far more time on our mattress than in our car.

When you go mattress shopping, wear shoes you can slip off easily, and lie on the mattresses you're checking out. Roll over. Spread out. Lie in the way you normally sleep—on your side, on your back, on your stomach. Don't go alone. Andrea Herman of the Better Sleep Council advises couples to shop together for a mattress. "The bottom line is finding a mattress that works for both of you," she says. Take your time. Lie on the mattress for at least 15 minutes when you're evaluating it. Oh, and try not to fall asleep!

Type. There are numerous types of mattresses available today. You can buy a mattress filled with water, air, or foam. The most popular type of mattress is an innerspring mattress, named for the coiled steel springs sandwiched between layers of padding. Today's innerspring mattresses have gotten thicker—between 9 and 15 inches, compared to the seven inches they used to be. The Swedish memory-foam mattresses, composed of a foam originally made for NASA astronauts, conform to your body imprint but come up under all your pressure points, with a thick, removable pillow top that can be laundered. Water beds these days are firmer than they used to be; the "waveless" water beds are specially designed so you don't get seasick every time your partner rolls over.

Frame. A high-quality bed frame ensures your mattress will last. A frame should have a rigid center support with a fifth leg and bed rails with at least ten wooden slats using a solid platform base with at least three rigid steel cross supports.

Cost. Prices for mattresses vary more than those for used cars, and the deals are just as negotiable, according to *Consumer Reports*. But in the end, the magazine learned that if you spend at least $450 for a twin-size mattress set, $600 for a full-size, $800 for a queen-size, and $1,000 for a king-size, you can get a quality, durable product.

Maintenance. Turn your mattress over and upside down every three months so you're sleeping on a less worn part.

Pillows

Your choice of a pillow can actually make a big difference in the quality of your sleep. A good pillow supports your head in natural alignment with your spine, thus providing you with a more comfortable, better night's sleep. But which type of pillow? Down? Synthetic? There's even one filled with buckwheat.

Or try water-filled. These pillows are like tiny water beds—you can adjust their firmness or softness depending on how much water you fill them with. Researchers at Johns Hopkins University in Baltimore tested three pillows—the subjects' usual pillow, a roll pillow, and a water-based pillow—on 41 men with benign back pain. The results? The water-based pillow provided a better night's sleep, with less pain. Such water-based pillows include the Chiroflow (*www.chiroflow.com*) and Mediflow (*www.pillowrx.com*).

Even if you don't want a water pillow, consider getting a new pillow. Pillows become worn out with all the wear and tear (and beating and thumping and flipping) they endure. With normal use and care, a natural-fill pillow (usually filled with down) can last up to 10 years. A synthetic pillow, on the other hand, lasts just a couple of years. Down is generally considered the best type of pillow, even for those with allergies. Look for pillows made with a patented process called "hyper clean" that removes any and all dust particles in the down. Choose your new pillow based on the position in which you start your night's sleep. As a rule of thumb it goes like this: medium for back sleepers, firm for side, and soft for stomach. Or just go with whatever gets you through the night.

Tonight: Try sleeping on a different pillow.

Later: Buy a water-based pillow and see if it improves your sleep.

Sheets and Blankets

Have you ever woken up in the middle of the night, unable to sleep because your sheets or mattress pad have come loose and twisted around your legs? Then you understand the importance of tight-fitting bedding. I'm on my third mattress pad for my one-year-old king-sized bed. I simply can't find one that stays tight, and the bumps and ripples make it difficult to fall back to sleep during middle-of-the-night insomnia attacks.

Treat yourself to some new sheets and, if necessary, a new mattress pad. Before you head for the store, measure the thickness of your mattress. As *Consumer Reports* discovered when its researchers tested sheets, even some sets that promise deep pockets didn't fit the magazine's 12½-inch-thick mattress. Some mattresses today are 15 or even 18 inches thick. Also, the higher the thread count (250 minimum), the softer the sheet.

Also consider using a comforter instead of a blanket. The lightness of a down comforter lying across you—compared to the tangled blankets that can result after a restless night—may improve your sleep. When buying a down comforter, you'll hear terms like "fill power." This just means how fluffy and puffy the comforter is. The higher the "fill power" the better the comforter and the longer it will last. Look for higher thread counts in the cover, resulting in a lighter, softer comforter, which also prevents the down "fill" from leaking to the outside air. This lightness also helps the fill to "puff up." The best down is Siberian down, the worst is duck feather, with goose and Hungarian down falling in the high middle.

> **Tonight.** Iron your sheets, first sprinkling them with a bit of lavender-scented water. Then make up your bed with the crisply ironed, fresh sheets.

> **Later.** Splurge and buy a set of high-quality, high-thread-count cotton sheets and a high-quality down comforter.

Room temperature

The temperature of your room is an important element in a good night's sleep, in terms of your ability both to fall asleep and to stay asleep. Sleep researchers say we sleep best at a temperature between 60 and 72 degrees F. Temperature is important because we lose some of our ability to regulate our body temperature during REM sleep, so abnormally hot or cold temperatures in the environment can disrupt this stage of sleep. Temperatures higher than 75, in particular, seem to reduce slow-wave and REM sleep.

> **Tonight:** Read over your checklist and your sleep diary and adjust the temperature in your room accordingly. If it's generally too warm and you don't have air-conditioning, switch to a cooler blanket or sleep with just a top sheet. If it's too cool, add an extra blanket instead of turning up the heat.

Light

Light, even short-term light that comes from turning on the bathroom light when you get up in the middle of the night, can interfere significantly enough with melatonin levels to make it difficult to fall back to sleep. One study found that being waked up and exposed to bright light at night can throw your biological clock off for a few days. Ambient light from street lights, cars, or neighbors' houses—even a full moon—that seeps through the slats in your blinds or around the edges of your shades or curtains might be one reason for your middle-of-the-night awakening. Your early-morning awakening might be due to the rising sun.

Tonight: Tack a heavy blanket over your window openings to seal out all traces of light. Put a dim night light in the bathroom and turn it on at night so you don't have to turn on the overhead light if you get up in the middle of the night.

Later: Buy blackout curtains. You can buy curtains that attach to the back of your regular curtains, so they look no different from the street. Also buy eyeshades that block the light.

Scent

Marcia Cronin follows a soothing ritual when she tucks her two daughters, 10 and 8, into bed. The 43-year-old sales consultant sprays some lavender scent on their pillows before kissing them good night. Tania Casselle, of Taos, New Mexico, puts a drop of lavender oil on her pillow. The scent, both women believe, helps induce sleep. They may be right. Victorian women routinely sniffed handkerchiefs dabbed with oil of lavender, and several studies have found essential oil of lavender can calm and soothe nearly as effectively as a tranquilizer. In one study, published in the British medical journal *Lancet*, researchers took nursing home patients off sedating drugs for two weeks, then infused the room with lavender oil. The patients slept just as well as they had with the sleeping pills.

Aromatherapy, which involves the use of essential oils such as lavender, relies on the direct connection of the olfactory nerve—which senses smell—and the brain; the olfactory nerve sends electrical messages directly into the limbic system, the part of the brain responsible for emotions, feelings, and moods. Because of this connection, essential oils can have effects on emotions and mental states, including memory, learning, emotions, thinking, and feeling.

> **Tonight:** Spray your bedroom and pillow with lavender scent. Light a lavender candle while you're lying in bed reading before you turn off your light (remember to blow out the candle before you go to sleep). And/or soak in a lavender-scented tub a few hours before bed.

Decor

What color is your bedroom? While a deep red works well for a dining room or living room, it could be overstimulating in your bedroom. Bedrooms should be peaceful, painted and decorated with pastels or other colors taken from nature—soothing creams or a pale mocha or sage green. Choose a color that makes you feel relaxed just by looking at it.

In addition to the color of your room, the accessories and mood you create can play a role in preparing you for sleep. Is your room cluttered and dirty? This can affect you as you try to go to sleep, making you feel anxious. Aim for a soothing environment, clear of clutter, clean, with smooth surfaces and items that appeal to you. For instance, put away any photographs, books, or mementos that remind you of unpleasant times in your life. Put a few plants in your bedroom. In addition to providing a soothing shot of green, they will also help humidify the air, which can lead to a better night's sleep.

> **Tonight:** Leaf through home magazines and paint chip samples searching for the perfect new color for your bedroom. Clear out any clutter in your room.

> **Later.** Paint your bedroom.

Noise

From the trucks and buses of the big city to the predawn chirping of birds in the spring and summer, sound is by far one of the primary reasons for a sleepless night or too-early awakening. Even sounds that fade into the background during the day—a running toilet, the cat licking herself, a houseguest with allergies—can leave you tossing and turning in the relative quiet of the night. One study conducted in Spain found that 9 percent of residents were forced to change the location of their bedroom as a result of noise, whereas another 11 percent were forced to sleep with the windows closed. In another study, 12 people living in areas of high traffic were studied to determine how the noise affected their sleep. Once their windows were double-glazed to reduce noise, they all slept better. Brain indications of deep sleep increased, and the subjects did better the next day on a test designed to measure drowsiness.

Ironically, even a lack of noise can disrupt your sleep, if, for instance, you're used to being lulled to sleep by the sounds of traffic.

Tonight:

Move your bed. Place it on the wall farthest from the window and, if possible, away from any wall adjacent to a room that has a lot of activity, e.g., the kitchen or family bathroom. **Use white noise.** Set your radio to the space between stations and turn the volume down. The soft static will provide a white noise to mask any other sounds. You can also buy a bubbling fountain—available even in drugstores these days—to produce a calming, soothing sound that serves to filter out more annoying noises. A fan or quiet air-conditioner can serve the same purpose. **Try earplugs.** The wax plugs that mold themselves to your ears are best. But make sure you aren't relying on your alarm to wake you up, or make sure it's set extra loud.

Later:

Check into having your windows double-glazed. Double-glazing significantly cuts sound transmission. Heavy drapes will also reduce noise. If you live in an apartment or condo above someone, consider carpeting your bedroom floor to provide another layer of soundproofing. Ask your landlord about carpeting the apartment above yours.

Create a Time-Free Zone

While you probably need an alarm clock to get you up in the morning (especially since you're probably suffering from sleep debt), having it face you all night as you lie in bed, or when you wake in the middle of the night and can't get back to sleep, will make things worse. Some insomniacs become obsessed with the time, staring at the slowly turning numbers on their digital clocks, growing more anxious with each minute.

Tonight: Put your clock under your bed, where you can hear it but won't see it.

Create a Sleep-Only Environment

Unless you live in a dorm room, where, by necessity, you also eat and work, your bedroom should be a work-free, stress-free zone. This means don't bring your work into bed with you, or your computer into your bedroom. Ideally, you shouldn't have a television in your room either. It's better to watch television in another room, and when it's time for sleep, make the physical change of moving into your bedroom. This tells your mind that it's time for sleep, not television watching.

This approach even has a name; it's called stimulus control. Basically, it helps you associate your bed with two things: sex and sleep (although I also associate mine with reading).

Tonight: Move the television, VCR, and computer out of your bedroom. Turn off the ringer on the phone.

Feeling Secure

How secure do you feel when you go to sleep? If you live in a rough neighborhood, make sure you have sturdy locks on your windows and doors, and, if possible an alarm system. You might also feel more secure if you can see the door of your room from the bed, or if your bed is placed away from a window. Have the phone within easy reach so you can call 911 if someone breaks in, and keep a can of pepper spray or mace within easy reach.

Tonight: Make the rounds of your house before you go to sleep to check that all doors and windows are closed and locked.

Later: Consider getting a burglar alarm or a dog.

Stop the Sneezing

Most bedding and mattresses are filled with dust mites and, if you've been sleeping with your windows open, pollen. The sneezing and congestion that results from allergic rhinitis is enough to keep even the most exhausted person awake.

Tonight: Wash all your bedclothes, including the mattress pad, in hot water before remaking your bed. Close all windows in your bedroom and sleep with the air conditioner on to reduce pollens.

Later: Consider a water bed. You can wipe down the bed every time you change your sheets, greatly eliminating a buildup of dust mites or mite dander. Also consider installing a wood floor or tile in your bedroom to reduce allergens from dust mites that hide in carpeting.

The Program: Day 1

Complete the bedroom evaluation and determine which areas of your room need work. Then, using the information provided throughout the rest of Day 1, redecorate and redesign your bedroom to ensure the best night's sleep possible.

Remember, the little things can make a big difference. In addition to the way in which you decorate your room and prepare your bed, make sure your room is "sleep-ready" when you turn out the lights. Keep the door shut if you have pets that wander through the house at night, and keep a night light on in the bathroom.

Now that you've got the right sleep environment, tomorrow we'll take a look at your presleep program.

DAY 2: THE PRESLEEP PROGRAM

Today you're going to develop your own presleep program—a series of steps that will help you prepare for sleep and banish the worries of the day. These behavioral modifications are highly effective. In one 1999 study that compared drug therapy and changing sleeping patterns over a two-year period, researchers found that behavioral changes produced the greatest improvements in sleep. Most of the participants who used the behavioral therapies no longer qualified as insomniacs. In contrast, half of those who took medication still had insomnia.

Review and Reflect

Look through your sleep diary, paying particular attention to the activities you engage in during the two hours before you get into bed. Keep those in mind as you read and work through the steps tonight and during the next week.

Limit Your Presleep Activities

While the vast majority of U.S. adults watch TV (87 percent) before they go to sleep, only 28 percent say that watching TV helps them fall asleep. In fact, most television can be too stimulating for a before-sleep activity. Turn the television off at least an hour before you go to sleep, and spend that hour either reading (which 53 percent of Americans do before sleeping) or practicing some of the relaxation techniques described below. Karen, of Phoenix, Arizona, switched from watching TV to doing crossword puzzles before going to bed, and found it helped focus her "ruminating" mind, enabling her to fall asleep much more quickly once she turned the light off.

To prepare your body for sleep, you might also try dimming the lights in the hour before you flip them off completely. The soft light will relax you and get you into "sleep mode."

Other don'ts before sleep tonight:

- Don't pay bills, check your work voice mail or E-mail, or tackle a complex project within the hour before bed. You're trying to relax, de-stress, and calm yourself. All of the above are nearly guaranteed to spike your blood pressure.
- Don't exercise less than three hours before you go to bed. For more on exercise and its effects on sleep, see Day 5 of the Seven-Day Sleep Program, page 114.

Tonight: Don't check your E-mail or voice mail after 7 p.m. Around 9 p.m., turn off the television set and settle in with a good book, your journal, or a calming hobby (needlepoint, model building, puzzles).

Time Your Presleep Bathing

"One remedy I try is washing my hair about 60 or 90 minutes before I want to sleep, then drying it with a hair dryer. The scalp massage, warm water, and warm air probably account for its helpfulness. Once your hair is dry, don't do anything aggravating that'll interfere with the relaxation. Just let yourself feel pleasantly groggy."
—Marie Shear, New York

Forget a before-bed shower. The force of the water is too energizing (that's why most of us shower in the morning even before that first cup of coffee). Instead, take a hot bath (as hot as you can stand it) two hours before bed. As your body cools, your temperature drops, a necessary physiological change if sleep is to occur. Don't take the bath too close to bedtime, however, or your body temperature will be too high to ensure instant sleep. You might also try pouring some oats into your bath; oats have a long history as a sleep aid (see Day 3).

Tonight: Take a hot bath laced with lavender oil and oats two hours before you go to sleep.

Understand and Embrace Your Presleep Ritual

"An important practical consideration is to have the light switch close enough that I don't have to move position to turn out the light. (I have a reading light attached to the headboard of the bed and the switch is right beside it.) I read until I'm about three-quarters asleep. I can reach up and turn out the light without actually being awake it seems. Usually in the morning I don't recall having turned out the light or put the bookmark in the book. If I turn out the light before I'm far enough asleep, that action wakes me and I have to turn the light back on and read again until I sleep. If I'm away from home and have to roll over to turn off a bedside lamp, the process of getting to sleep can be prolonged."
   —Diane, Minneapolis, Minn.

My own presleep routine goes like this: Turn off computer and lights, let the dog out one last time, walk through the house turning out lights, put the dog in with my son (who seems to have no problems sleeping with or without a pet), change into my nightgown, wash and cream my face, brush my teeth, use the toilet, fill my water glass, slide into bed with a deep sigh, and open my book.

As I perform each of these actions, my brain receives a

message: It's time for sleep. I'm conditioning myself to go to sleep. That last step—reading a book—is critical. No matter how exhausted I am, if I don't read for at least five or ten minutes, usually half an hour, I can't fall asleep.

Everyone has their own presleep rituals, even dogs, who sniff, walk around in a circle a few times, then curl up. My children refuse to go to sleep without their good-night story, their closet light on, a book-on-tape playing, and their stuffed animals surrounding them (plus a good-night kiss). Charles Dickens made sure that, in whichever bed he slept in, his head pointed north and his feet south so the earth's electromagnetic currents would flow through his body, enhancing his sleep.

In one study of 90 people with normal sleep habits, everyone went to the bathroom before going to bed; 25 percent had a snack or light meal in the two-hour period before bed; 60 percent set an alarm, and 27 percent had a bath or shower. Twenty-three percent checked the door locks or windows, and 49 percent read in bed. Nine percent slept with a cat on the bed.

What's your ritual like? Tonight, as you move through the steps of your sleep ritual, try to be mindful of what you're doing, reminding yourself that with each step, you're preparing yourself for sleep, not just taking out the garbage or folding that last load of laundry. On the other hand, if you're a chronic insomniac and your rituals only serve to remind you that you're going to have trouble falling asleep, find new rituals.

Tonight: Pay attention to your presleep ritual, and write it down in your sleep diary before you go to bed, if you haven't already done so.

Watch Your Reading Material

While I'm a big proponent of reading before sleep, make sure the book you're reading isn't too stimulating (like the latest Stephen King thriller or a murder mystery). I remember reading King's *The Shining* late one night, and being so terrified I couldn't turn my light off for hours. Another problem arises if the book you're reading is too engrossing that you simply can't put it down. Next thing you know, it's 2 a.m., and, tired as you are, you lie there worrying about the sleep you missed and your early morning meeting. One suggestion: Purchase a light that simulates a sunset, starting out bright then gradually dimming to full dark. Once it's too dim to read, you'll know it's time to put the book down. These lights can be found at Rise & Shine Natural Alarm Clock Lamps from Verilux, 888-236-7231.

Tonight: Try reading a book of poetry or short stories before bed.

Keep a Journal

Every night, before I turn off my computer for the evening, I redo my daily to-do list. Once my list of tasks are on paper, they stop making me tense and anxious. You can do this yourself as a way of "downloading" the stresses of the day. As part of your presleep ritual tonight, spend ten minutes either making a list of things you're worried/stressed/anxious about, including a to-do list, or just quietly writing your thoughts about the day in a journal. Once you put the pen down, mentally close the lid on that group of worries. You don't have to worry you'll forget them—you have them in writing—and they won't keep you awake, either.

Tonight: Spent 15 minutes writing the worries of the day in your journal before you get into bed.

Reconsider Sex

Contrary to what you might think, sex is actually *not* the best activity to engage in just before sleep. Even after orgasm, your body is still aroused, much the same way it would be if you'd just done 15 push-ups before bed, or gone for a brisk walk. If the sex doesn't go well, you're adding stress to the equation. Women, in particular, seem to have problems falling asleep after sex, says Dr. Joyce Walsleben. In her book *A Woman's Guide to Sleep*, she notes that women tend to remain at a higher level of arousal after a climax. This may be related to high levels of the stress hormone norepinephrine, which prevents you from falling asleep.

Every individual is different and sex does release endorphins, chemicals which contribute to a sense of well-being. In one of the few studies that have tried to examine this issue (in which participants masturbated before falling asleep), subjects fell asleep in the same length of time whether they reached orgasm or not.

If you're having problems falling asleep, and you typically have intercourse before you go to sleep, try abstinence for a few nights, then check your sleep diary and see if it makes any difference. Human's sexual hormones—the ones that contribute to arousal—are typically higher in the early morning, anyway.

Tonight: Explain to your partner that you are trying to identify presleep actions that may be interfering with your sleep, and ask him/her to understand your need to abstain from before-sleep sex. Or, you could surprise your partner with before-dinner lovemaking!

Warm Your Feet

Recent studies suggest that inadequate dilation of your blood vessels may cause some sleep problems, says Dr. Walsleben. That's because when you lie down, your core temperature drops, and heat is redistributed to your arms and legs via dilated blood vessels. If you're cold, your blood vessels won't dilate because they are trying to keep closer to your core body.

Tonight: Dig out your hiking socks and slip them on before bed, or snuggle a hot water bottle between your feet.

Dress for Sleep

What do you wear to sleep? Maybe you sleep in the nude, or in a Victoria's Secret silk slip of a nightgown. Whatever you wear, always go for cooler rather than warmer, since your body temperature rises during the night. If you get too warm, it could wake you up. For women moving into menopause and experiencing hot flashes, choose cotton sleeping clothes if you choose anything; the fabric breathes and will keep you cooler.

Tonight: Sleep in something different from what you typically sleep in. If you usually sleep in the nude, try a light T-shirt; if you generally sleep in flannel, try sleeping in the nude. See if it makes any difference.

Think Your Way to Sleep

Experts say that sleep is easily influenced by the power of suggestion. In one 1985 study, volunteers were offered $25 if they could fall asleep quickly. Participants took twice as long to fall asleep as a control group who weren't receiving any reward. So if you think you can't fall asleep, you won't fall asleep. Conversely, if you climb into bed certain you're going to drift off within a few minutes, you're more likely to do just that.

Tonight, as you're brushing your teeth and washing your face, keep repeating the following: "I am going to fall asleep quickly tonight. I am going to fall asleep quickly tonight." Visualize yourself sleeping soundly, the peacefulness of the quiet room, and your steady, deep breathing. If, after lying in bed for 15 or 20 minutes, you still can't sleep, get up. The longer you lie there, the more upset you'll become about your inability to fall asleep and the less likely it is that you'll actually fall asleep. Instead, turn on a soft light and read, listen to music, or write in your journal. Try to stay awake. Then, just like the participants in the experiment described above, you'll be more likely to fall asleep.

Peter Hauri, Ph.D., coauthor of *No More Sleepless Nights* (John Wiley and Sons, 1996) and director of the Mayo Clinic Sleep Program, suggests you look at this time as "extra" time you can spend doing something you enjoy, things you might not otherwise have the time to do.

As with every suggestion provided throughout this book, keep in mind that your own individuality may require a different approach. For instance, Alisa Bauman, of Emmaus, Pennsylvania, says this advice never works for her. "For one, the bed is comfortable. I'd rather be in bed than doing something else. Two, my husband is asleep, so I don't usually want to wake him up. Three, it always takes me 30 minutes to an hour to fall asleep. If I got up every ten minutes, I'd be up all night."

Tonight: Give yourself permission to turn the light back on if you haven't fallen asleep within 20 minutes, rather than tossing and turning another 40.

Meditate Your Way to Sleep

Many of us who are in sleep debt find it difficult to meditate during the day because we have a tendency to fall asleep. Now's the time to take advantage of that "problem" and meditate yourself to sleep. Here's how:

1. Climb into bed and arrange yourself in your customary sleeping position.
2. Once you're comfortable, close your eyes.
3. Visualize yourself walking down a staircase. With each step you descend, say the word "sleep" in your mind, like a mantra. As you descend each step, feel the tension lift just a bit more from your neck, your arms, your legs. This staircase is infinite, but by the time you reach the bottom step, you should be asleep.

If you can manage to meditate during the day, try it. One study of eight women found that those who meditated regularly had higher nighttime levels of the sleep hormone melatonin than those who didn't.

Tonight: Use this visualization exercise to help you fall asleep.

Treat Yourself Like a Child

For writer Tania Casselle, a good night story helps her get to sleep. "When I was living alone," she says, "I often taped radio plays or stories that were broadcast in the day, and played them back at low volume. Probably because my mind stopped working on all the events of the day and everything I had to do tomorrow, just to concentrate on listening to the story, they were perfect for lulling me off to sleep. I always had to rewind the next night to just a few minutes on from where I started the night before. Now that I'm married, I ask my husband to tell me a story if I'm really stuck. He rarely gets more than two minutes into his tale before I am snoozing. . . ."

Try books on tape for the same effects. My, 9-year-old always falls asleep listening to one of his Harry Potter books on tape.

> **Tonight:** Slip a book on tape (or CD) into your portable stereo and fall asleep to the soothing sounds of someone reading aloud.

Retrain Your Bladder

As we age, middle-of-the-night bathroom trips provide one of the most common reasons for interrupted sleep. In men, it's often an aging prostate sending the signal to urinate; in women, it's bladder incontinence caused by dropping estrogen levels or pregnancy.

To minimize middle-of-the-night awakenings:

- Don't drink anything for at least an hour (preferably two) before sleep.

- Retrain your bladder: Start voiding on a very strict schedule during the day, like every two hours, then resist any urge to void until the next scheduled time. By doing this over several weeks, your bladder starts to listen to your brain. Gradually increase the time between voiding.
- If this doesn't work, talk to your doctor about some of the newer medications for overactive bladder, like Detrol (tolterodine) and Ditropan (oxybutynin chloride).

Tonight: If middle-of-the-night urinations are part of your sleep problem, don't drink anything for at least an hour before you fall asleep.

Engage in Massage

I think massage is the most underrated health technique we have in the twenty-first century. I find it helpful for everything from pain and soreness to depression and insomnia. While it's doubtful you'll be able to find a massage therapist to come to your home at 11 p.m., if you sleep with someone ask him/her to give you a massage (promise your partner a midafternoon massage on the weekend in return). Keep some scented massage oil by your bed, and have your partners work out the tensions. If you live or sleep alone, try a self-massage. Gently move your fingers in a firm, circular motion around your forehead, eyes, temples, neck, and shoulders, taking deep breaths in and out as you do so.

Tonight: Give your partner an IOU coupon for a massage at a future date, hand him/her the bottle of massage oil, and turn over on your stomach.

Have a Mentally Active Day

Studies find that poor sleepers often spend more time in their day sitting around, shopping, or watching TV, rather than in activities that engage their minds. This is particularly common in people who have retired, or home-makers whose children have left home. While exercise is important (more on that in Day 5 of the program), engaging your mind is just as important. Consider taking classes, volunteering, or pursuing a hobby. Take up cross-word puzzles, research your genealogy, become a Master Gardener.

Today: Do something you've never (or rarely) done before. Visit a museum, pull out your old oil painting equipment and begin a new painting, plant (or plan) a garden. As you're trying to fall asleep, replay the activity and the satisfaction it gave you in your mind.

Go to Bed at the Same Time

Read any magazine article about insomnia and sleep and one of the first pieces of advice the writer gives is to go to bed at the same time every night. Dr. Dement believes so strongly in this advice that he's been known to leave dinner parties early—even when he's the host—to make his 9 p.m. bedtime. Keeping to a regular schedule gets you in the mindset for sleep the same time every night.

Starting tonight, go to bed at the same time for a week. Then review your sleep diary and see if it's making any difference.

Tonight: Decide what time you're going to make your "regular" bedtime and climb into bed at the appointed hour.

Try Stress-Reduction Mechanisms

Deep breathing. Ever watch a baby breathe? His belly pooches out with each inhalation; his chest and belly sink with each exhalation. He's breathing the way nature intended. We adults, on the other hand, are shallow breathers, barely taking in enough oxygen to maintain adequate oxygen/carbon dioxide levels. This, in turn, starves our body of oxygen. Too little oxygen might cause you to hyperventilate. Your heart beats faster to pump more blood, your lungs and kidneys start working overtime, and your blood vessels constrict, turning your hands ice-cold.

Breathing correctly is so beneficial (it's been linked to lower blood pressure, reduced levels of heart disease, even your overall life span) that some people even hire breathing coaches.

You probably don't need a coach. Just follow this simple exercise:

1. Lie on your back in bed, and put a hand on your stomach.
2. Breathe in from your diaphragm to the count of 3. You'll know you're breathing in from your diaphragm if you see your hand rise.
3. Exhale slowly, to the count of 3. Watch your hand go down.
4. Repeat until you fall asleep.
5. For an added boost, allow a brief moan to escape through your mouth with each exhalation. Picture your stress escaping with each moan.

Visualization. In this relaxation exercise, lie on your back in bed in the dark, close your eyes, and picture a moment in your life when you felt deep relaxation. Maybe it was that mid-winter break you took in the islands, lying on the white-hot sand, the sun beating down on you, the scent of coconut oil in the air, an icy drink by your side, and the knowledge of a sumptuous dinner to come. Don't just see the picture—feel the heat of the sun, smell the suntan lotion, hear the crashing waves. With any luck, your vision will follow you into your dreams.

You can also visualize your way to sleep. Norman Ford, author of 75 *Proven Ways to Get a Good Night's Sleep* (Prentice Hall, 1994), suggests you "ride the elevator down" into sleep, with your relaxation deepening with every floor you see lit on the indicator. He also recommends the "counting to zero" visualization, in which you visualize a large figure 9 glowing brightly green. As you watch it fade, your tension fades with it. Then you visualize a large, glowing 8, and watch it fade, too. Continue until you reach zero.

Progressive relaxation. This exercise works to rid your body of the tension stored in your muscles. Start by tensing your toes, then relaxing. Then tense your foot, relax. Tense your calf muscles, relax. Continue in this manner as you work your way up your body, tensing then relaxing each muscle in turn until you reach the muscles that govern your forehead (if you're not already asleep).

The Program: Day 2

Make a list of every activity you currently do before you go to bed. Compare it to the recommended activities in this section. Abandon any part of your old routine that seems ineffective and instead, try out three new presleep activities each night until you find a program that works for you.

Tomorrow, we'll explore some teas, tonics, and tablets to help coax sleep along.

DAY 3: TEAS, TONICS, AND OTHER NATURAL SLEEP REMEDIES

Today, more than 242 million Americans use some form of dietary supplement—vitamins, minerals, herbal remedies, or specialty supplement—as a safe and natural way to maintain good health and supplement inadequate diets. Many of these supplements are an aid to getting a good night's sleep. In fact, natural sleep remedies have been passed down through folk medicine for thousands of years, emerging today as one of the strongest categories of herbal and alternative medicine. Almost one out of five adults use herbal remedies (18 percent) when they have problems sleeping. It makes sense since, unlike the over-the-counter and prescription medications described in Chapter 2, herbal and other natural remedies are usually gentler and don't leave you with a sleep "hangover."

Herbal medicines are made solely from parts of whole plants—e.g., leaves, bark, or roots—in contrast to conventional modern medicines that extract and concentrate specific constituents. Herbal medicines are believed to be effective, yet without side effects, because the basic parts of the plant act to balance the effects of the active ingredient within the body.

Still, just because something is "natural" doesn't mean it's entirely safe. And, since the Food and Drug Administration doesn't oversee the quality of natural supplements, nor confirm manufacturer claims, this is an instance in which the consumer must take care. Don't take any herbal medications or natural supplements without considering potential interactions with other medications you're taking. And always let your health provider know everything you take—even vitamins.

Be patient; many natural remedies require several days, weeks, or even months, before their effects are felt. That's far different from the nearly immediate benefit of prescription medications. And always follow package dosing directions. More is *not* necessarily better.

As part of Day 3 of the Seven-Day Sleep Program, you're going to learn what's available in terms of natural sleep aids, what works, what doesn't, and what the potential dangers are, if any.

Herbs and Teas

A tincture is an extract, usually herbal, usually made with a mixture of water and alcohol. A tea is made by pouring boiling water over an herb and letting it steep.

Catnip

This herb quiets your nervous system and relaxes your muscles. It also contains nepetalactone, a mild sedative.

What the studies show. There are no available clinical studies.

Recommended dosage: Experts recommend you steep 1 heaping teaspoon of dried herbs per cup of hot water and drink it one hour before bed. Or take 30 to 40 drops of tincture two or three times a day. For a better taste, combine it with lemon balm and chamomile.

Chamomile

Chamomile tea has been used for centuries as a sleep aid and relaxant. It's readily available on your grocery store shelves and is perfectly safe.

What the studies show: When 12 patients who'd had a ventricular catheterization, a painful procedure in which a tube is inserted through a main artery to observe the health of that artery, received chamomile tea after the procedure, 10 of the 12 fell into a deep sleep.

Recommended dosage: Experts recommend one cup an hour before bed.

Warning: If you're allergic to ragweed, you may also be allergic to chamomile.

Dill

The word "dill" comes from the Norse "dilla," meaning "to lull," and folk remedies say this herb is an insomnia cure.

What the studies show: There are no available clinical studies.

Recommended dosage: Experts recommend using dill to make a tea. Pour 1 cup of boiling water over 1 teaspoon of crushed dill seeds, steep for 10 minutes, strain, and drink one hour before bed.

California Poppy

This herb helps induce sleep by affecting transmission of various neurotransmitters, chemicals in your brain.

What the studies show. There are no available clinical studies.

Recommended dosage: Experts recommend a 2-to-4-milliliter tincture or two capsules before bed.

Jamaica Dogwood

This herb is calming, easing pain and disturbing persistent thoughts, which are often causes of insomnia.

What the studies show: There are no available clinical studies.

Recommended dosage: As a tincture, experts recommend 5 to 20 drops.

Hops

Hops, an essential ingredient in beer, contains the relaxant isovaleric acid, also found in valerian. Try a glass of nonalcoholic beer, which is made with hops but contains no alcohol to interfere with your sleep, or a supplement.

What the studies show: In one German study comparing a benzodiazepine and a hops/valerian preparation, both contributed equally to sleep quality, although participants experienced withdrawal symptoms with the benzodiazepine.

Recommended dosage. Experts recommend 0.5 grams of the dried herb, or its equivalent in extract, taken one to several times a day.

Warnings. Not recommended for pregnant women or women with estrogen-dependent breast cancer.

Kava

Kava (or kava-kava) is known for its calming effect on the nervous system, acting on your brain similarly to the way benzodiazepines like Valium work.

What the studies show: One British study of 24 patients suffering from stress-induced insomnia were treated for six weeks with 120 milligrams of kava, followed by two weeks off treatment, then 19 of the remaining patients received 600 milligrams of valerian daily for another six weeks. Overall, the participants' total stress was significantly reduced, as was their insomnia. The main side effect was "vivid dreams" with valerian (16 percent of participants) followed by 12 percent who had some dizziness.

Recommended dosage: Using capsules standardized to 30 percent kavalactones, experts recommend 70 to 210 milligrams a day.

Warning: Extended use or high doses may cause liver damage. Don't take with alcohol or barbiturates or other sleep aids, or if you're driving or operating heavy machinery.

Lemon Balm

In ancient times, lemon balm was viewed as the ultimate remedy for a troubled nervous system. Today, it's used to calm nerves, aiding in insomnia. Lemon balm's actions are due largely to chemicals called terpenes.

What the studies show: When valerian and lemon balm were tested against Halcion, a prescription insomnia drug, the valerian/lemon balm combo matched the prescription counterpart in its ability to induce sleep and affect the quality of sleep. The big difference was felt the next day: Those taking the prescription reported feeling "hung over" and had trouble concentrating, while those taking the herbal remedy reported no next-day side effects.

Recommended dosage: Experts recommend 1.5 to 4.5 grams of lemon balm in a tea before bed.

Lettuce

The ancient Greeks believed that lettuce induced sleep, so they often served a lettuce soup at the end of a meal. However, one Roman emperor served it at the beginning of his feasts so he could torture his guests by forcing them to stay awake in his presence. Even the Flopsy bunnies in Beatrix Potter's works fall into such a deep sleep after eating lettuce that their enemy catches them unawares.

What the studies show: Although there are no available clinical studies on lettuce and sleep, the vegetable does contain a sleep-inducing substance called "lecturcarium," which has effects similar to opium without that drug's stimulant effects. Lettuce also contains an anticramping agent called hyoscyarnin, which helps relax muscles.

Recommended dosage: Experts recommend making lettuce tea. To make it, simmer 3 to 4 large lettuce leaves in ½ cup of water for 15 minutes, then remove from heat and add 2 sprigs of fresh mint (to disguise the bitterness of the lettuce brew). Steep for 5 minutes, strain, and drink half an hour before bed.

Oats

Folk remedies call for oats as a sleep aid and nerve tonic, and in modern times they've been found to be useful for stress, jet lag, or sleeping pill withdrawal.

What the studies show. There are no available clinical trials.

Recommended dosage: Experts recommend making a tea with 1 heaping tablespoon (approximately 15 grams) of oats brewed with 1 cup of boiling water. As a tincture, oats are often taken at ½ to 1 teaspoon (3 to 5 milliliters) three times per day. They are also available as capsules or tablets, and you can take 1 to 4 grams per day. Or try bathing in oats dissolved in hot water.

Passionflower

This herb was used by the Aztecs as a sedative and pain reliever. Along with valerian and chamomile, its active ingredients bind to the same brain receptors as benzodiazepine medications like Valium.

What the studies show: There are no published studies in humans on the effects of passionflower on insomnia. However, passionflower significantly prolonged sleeping time in rats.

Recommended dosage: Experts recommend drinking a cup of passionflower tea (4 to 8 grams of the herb) or taking 20 to 40 drops of the tincture in water half an hour before bed.

Skullcap

This Chinese herb has been used for thousands of years for the treatment of pain and insomnia.

What the studies show: There are no available clinical studies.

Recommended dosage: Experts recommend drinking a cup of skullcap tea (1 teaspoon of skullcap in 1 cup of boiling water) before bed. It blends well with other calming herbs such as lemon balm, catnip, chamomile, and linden flowers.

Valerian

This herb is the most widely used sleep aid in Europe and one of the best-selling herbs in America. Its use as a sleep aid dates back a thousand years, and the U.S. Food and Drug Administration rates valerian as GRAS (generally recognized as safe).

What the studies show: In one well-designed study of 128 volunteers who took 400 milligrams of valerian extract at bedtime, the volunteers reported that they fell asleep quicker, slept better, and woke up fewer times in the night.

Recommended dosage: Valerian can be taken as a tea, a tablet, or in tincture form, and can both shorten the time it takes to fall asleep and improve your sleep without side effects. Experts recommend 20 to 60 drops of tincture or 300 to 500 milligrams of a capsule of concentrated extract standardized to contain at least 0.5 percent valerenic acid half an hour before bed each day.

Warnings: Don't take valerian during the day, and don't use it with any other sleep- or mood-enhancing drugs. Don't take valerian over long periods of time; you may experience withdrawal symptoms.

How to Make an Herbal Tea

Pour 1 cup of boiling water over 1 to 3 teaspoons of the dried herb. Let steep at least 5 minutes, strain, let cool slightly, then drink.

Supplements

Melatonin

This hormone, secreted by the pineal gland, plays a critical role in sleep, as described in Chapter 2. In very low doses (up to 0.5 milligrams), melatonin can shift your biological clock, enabling you to get to sleep earlier than your normal bedtime. That's why travelers often use it to lessen the effects of jet lag and shift work.

What the studies show: Several studies show that melatonin is effective. In one, night shift workers used either melatonin or a placebo on their nights off (when they typically have trouble falling asleep). The melatonin increased their overall sleep quality. In another study it improved the quality of sleep for elderly patients with insomnia. Still, researchers note that long-term studies are needed.

Recommended dosage: While most over-the-counter melatonin supplements come in doses of 3 milligrams, experts recommend starting lower, at 0.5 milligrams, and building up. If you're groggy in the morning, reduce the amount. Don't ever take more than 10 milligrams. Try taking it 30 minutes before you go to bed.

Warnings: Don't take melatonin if you have heart disease. Side effects in clinical trials include headache, depression, tachycardia (racing heart), and itching. There is also some evidence it may affect human sperm and egg cells, as well as the human reproductive cycle. Don't take it if you're pregnant or breast-feeding, under age 35, have a blood or immune system cancer, or have kidney disease.

5-hydroxytryptophan (5-HTP)

5-HTP is a precursor to L-tryptophan, an amino acid found in plants and animals that we get from our diets, and L-tryptophan is a precursor to serotonin, a hormone that plays a major role in our sleep cycles.

What the studies show: Several double-blind clinical studies have found that 5-HTP helps participants fall asleep quicker and stay asleep longer. It also increases REM sleep and deep-sleep stages 3 and 4, without increasing overall sleep.

Recommended dosage: Experts recommend taking this supplement according to package directions. To increase the sedative effects of 5-HTP, take it with a food high in carbohydrates, such as fruit or fruit juice, near bedtime.

Warnings: 5-HTP may interact with certain antidepressants (including selective serotonin reuptake inhibitors

[SSRIs] like Prozac, and monoamine oxidase inhibitors [MAOIs]), causing serious negative side effects. Reports of eosinophilia-myalgia syndrome, which killed 39 people in 1989 who took contaminated L-tryptophan, occasionally surface with 5-HTP.

Alternative Therapies for Insomnia

Chiropractic

You wouldn't think aligning your spine would help you sleep better, but some people claim it helps. Although there are no studies on the effects of chiropractic and sleep, neck problems can sometimes cause sleep-disrupting tension and anxiety. Chiropractic treatment can relieve these symptoms.

Acupuncture

Reports in the medical literature suggest that acupuncture, in which very fine needles are inserted into certain points in your body to release chi, the body's life energy, is nearly 90 percent successful in treating insomnia. In one study, acupuncture used to treat patients with HIV/AIDS significantly improved participants' ability to sleep as well as their sleep quality after five weeks of treatment. Researchers think that sites on the central nervous system that receive acupuncture signals are also involved in the regulation of the sleep/wake cycles. Can't stand needles? Consider acupressure, or shiatsu, in which practitioners work with the same points used in acupuncture, stimulating these sites with finger pressure instead of inserting needles.

The Program: Day 3

Tonight's program is very simple: Thirty minutes before bed, brew a cup of chamomile tea. Try a different herbal tea or extract every night for the next week, making sure to track the results in your sleep diary so you can see which herb works best for you. If you need additional help falling and staying asleep, consult with your doctor before trying melatonin and 5-HTP.

Tomorrow: Eating your way to sleep.

DAY 4: EATING TO SLEEP

In the comic strip *Blondie*, Dagwood is forever whipping up mammoth sandwiches and snacks stuffed with stomach-searing ingredients, then nonchalantly heading up to bed where he sleeps like a baby. In real life, however, he'd lie in bed for hours, his stomach roiling like the deck of a ship in a storm, or drift off, only to be awakened by a terrible thirst, a need to urinate, or a horrible nightmare. For in real life—which rarely mimics a comic strip—what you eat and when you eat it determines the length and quality of your sleep.

Conversely, how well you sleep also determines how much you eat, since studies find that people with a chronic lack of sleep tend to eat more, particularly more high-fat foods. Another link between appetite and sleep is that the less deep sleep you get, the more weight you seem to gain. Researchers at the University of Chicago found that the less deep sleep (stage 3 and 4) subjects got, the less growth hormone they released, all of which is associated with increased fat and abdominal obesity, reduced muscle mass and strength, and reduced ability to exercise.

Review and Reflect

Today you're going to take a long, hard look at what you eat, when you eat it, even where you eat it to determine what role, if any, your diet plays in your insomnia. First, take a few minutes to review your sleep diary, paying particular attention to what you ate and drank on the days you had trouble falling asleep and those when you slept fine. See a pattern? Make a list of the foods you consumed on the insomnia days, and begin eliminating them one-by-one from your diet, tracking how you sleep each night you go without.

Later, we'll suggest a meal plan especially designed to get you sleeping tonight.

Do What Works for You

It's important to remember that, as with all recommendations throughout this book, what works for one person may not work for you. For instance, Marie Shear of New York says she finds half a pint of ice cream or sorbet, or a piece of cake or pie, the perfect antidote to insomnia, even though she admits it has a couple of disadvantages: "One, you end up looking like the Goodyear blimp. Two, my reaction to sugar may be atypical, since sugar is generally considered a stimulant, not a sedative."

Marie is right: Sugar is a stimulant, but a very short-acting stimulant. Marie may be reacting to the blood-sugar crash that occurs about an hour after eating such a sweet meal. She also has no problems with caffeine, noting: "It neither gives me a lift when I want one or keeps me awake when I want to sleep. So my own chemistry may be out of whack." Her chemistry probably isn't "out of whack," just different from other people's. Yours may differ, too. So if, for example, you find upon reading your sleep diary that your typical post-dinner cup of coffee has no effect on your sleep (i.e., you cut it out for a few days and still had trouble sleeping), then by all means reintroduce it.

Follow a Healthy Diet

Americans' nutritional habits need a major overhaul. Our diets are filled with processed foods and empty calories, and are high in fat and sodium. It's not easy to eat healthy in our world of drive-through and microwaved meals. Even nutritionists have a difficult time putting together healthy diets. When nutritionists in one study were charged with coming up with menus designed to meet the Dietary Guidelines for Americans, only 11 of 53 met the Recommended Daily Allowances (RDA) for zinc, half were deficient in vitamin B_6, and one-third lacked enough iron.

If you're deliberately dieting, or you're a vegetarian, you may have even more serious vitamin deficiencies. This is important, because even marginal vitamin deficiencies can cause insomnia. That's why it's so important to follow a healthy diet. It's important to eat lots of fruits and vegetables, lean meats and poultry, whole grains (try whole wheat pastas for a nutty, chewy treat), and stay away from high-fat foods (all fast foods) and animal fats, such as butter.

The American Heart Association recommends the following healthy diet. Following this diet will not only help ensure a good night's sleep, it will also help reduce your risk for a heart attack, stroke, and cancer, and help you drop a few pounds as well.

Eat a variety of fruits and vegetables. Choose five or more servings per day. If you find this difficult, find ways to "hide" fruits and vegetables. For instance, add prepackaged grated carrots to spaghetti sauce. Slice up a banana on your morning cereal. Add two slices of tomato and lettuce to every lunchtime sandwich. Even the garlic and onions you use to flavor a dish during cooking count.

Eat a variety of grain products, including whole grains. Choose six or more servings per day. This means choosing brown rice over white, whole wheat bread over white, interesting grains like barley and quinoa, and high-fiber cereals instead of those loaded with sugar.

Include fat-free and low-fat milk products, fish, legumes (beans), skinless poultry, and lean meats. Make meat the side dish on your plate instead of the main dish. Always make sure more of your plate is covered with vegetables, fruits, and whole grains than with the meat itself.

Choose the right fats and oils. This means opting for olive or canola oil, instead of solid fats like butter, margarine, or shortening, which contain artery-clogging saturated fats.

Balance calories in with calories out. To find that number, multiply the number of pounds you weigh now by 15. This represents the average number of calories used in one day if you're moderately active. If you get very little exercise, multiply your weight by 13 instead of 15. Less-active people burn fewer calories.

Limit nutritionally empty foods. Soft drinks, candy, and other sweets are high in calories, but low in nutrition. Try to cut them out.

Limit foods high in saturated fat, trans fat, and/or cholesterol. These include full-fat milk products, fatty meats, tropical oils, partially hydrogenated vegetable oils, and egg yolks.

Limit salt. Get less than 6 grams of salt per day (2,400 milligrams of sodium). Learn to read labels. Many canned and processed foods are loaded with sodium.

Watch the alcohol. The American Heart Association recommends you have no more than one alcoholic drink per day if you're a woman and no more than two if you're a man. "One drink" means it has no more than ½ ounce of pure alcohol. Examples of one drink are 12 ounces of beer, 4 ounces of wine, 1½ ounces of 80-proof spirits or 1 ounce of 100-proof spirits.

Vitamins and Minerals That Affect Sleep

Get vitamins and minerals through food

Although you can buy a supplement to replace nearly every nutrient identified in food, the best way to get vitamins, minerals and other nutrients is still the old-fashioned way—through food.

Calcium/Magnesium

"A combination calcium/magnesium tablet, taken about a half hour before I want to go to sleep, usually helps me."
   —Carol Sorgen, Baltimore, Md.

Carol has discovered on her own one of the best-kept sleep aid secrets. Calcium and magnesium—both of which play a role in nearly every physiological process of your body—also play a role in sleep. Calcium, for instance, helps regulate muscle movements, and tense muscles can keep you up at night. A deficiency in both minerals can lead to leg cramps. Yet nearly half of all Americans are deficient in calcium.

Magnesium, the fourth most abundant element in the brain, is also a natural sedative, essential in regulating your central nervous system and soothing excitability. Studies show that people who are severely lacking in this essential element find they experience epilepsy-type convulsions, dizziness, and muscle tremors or twitching, as well as irritability, anxiety, confusion, depression, apathy, loss of appetite, and insomnia. But, as the USDA notes, you don't have to be severely deficient in magnesium for your brain to become hyperactive (and a hyperactive brain is not the best state for a good night's sleep).

In one six-month study, USDA researchers had 13 women consume 115 milligrams of magnesium daily—or about 40 percent of the Recommended Dietary Allowance (RDA)—for three months. Then for the next three months, they got 315 milligrams daily—a little more than the 280 milligrams recommended for women. After only six weeks of marginal intake, they had significant differences in brain function. Even a marginal deficiency in magnesium excited the brain's neurons, the USDA notes. Another study found that magnesium supplements reduced the time it took people with insomnia to fall asleep, their number of nighttime awakenings, and their daytime anxiety and tension.

In yet another study, people who complained of constant fatigue increased their strength and energy within five to ten days after they started taking magnesium and potassium supplements, while yet another study found such supplements helped 75 of 80 participants to sleep better and awaken more refreshed. So experts recommend taking a mineral supplement containing 600 milligrams calcium with 300 milligrams magnesium just before bed.

Good food sources: Good sources of magnesium include whole grains, nuts, peanut butter, cottonseed, peanut and soybean flours, green leafy vegetables, and spices. Good sources of calcium include low- and nonfat dairy, calcium-fortified soy products, leafy green vegetables, green beans, broccoli, blackstrap molasses, and sardines with bones.

The B Vitamins

Many of the B vitamins play an important role in sleep and energy. Many Americans are deficient in these important vitamins, particularly women who take birth control pills. If you supplement, don't take Bs on their own; it's always best to take B vitamins together. Experts recommend one B complex supplement, 50 to 100 milligrams, every morning, even if you're sleeping fine. Among the specific B vitamins that affect sleep:

Thiamin (B_1). Thiamin helps convert carbohydrates in food into energy, promotes healthy nerves, and enhances mood. People with insomnia often have low levels of thiamin. In one study of older people, those with low thiamin levels who received thiamin supplements found their sleep and energy improved. The supplements also lowered their blood pressure and weight. Older people are more prone to thiamin deficiencies than other age groups.

Good food sources:	Asparagus, pork, fresh mussels, sunflower seeds, brazil nuts, salmon, pasta, wheat, avocados, oats, rice, soy milk, and barley.

Pyridoxine (B_6). This vitamin stimulates the pineal gland to secrete increased amounts of melatonin. It's also required for the conversion of the amino acid tryptophan to serotonin. In fact, one sign of inadequate vitamin B_6 is the inability to dream or recall dreams. Too much, and you may have dreams so vivid you're exhausted in the morning. Early in this century, mental hospitals were full of "hopelessly ill" patients whose mental confusion and agitation were the result of severe vitamin B deficiencies.

Good food sources: Cereals, beans, meat, poultry, fish, and some fruits and vegetables.

Niacin (B_3). This vitamin helps in the transformation of the amino acid tryptophan into serotonin, thus helping regulate production of melatonin and the sleep/wake cycle. Studies also find that niacin can improve REM sleep and decrease the amount of time people with insomnia spend awake, particularly for insomniacs who wake up in the middle of the night.

Good food sources: Most meats.

Cobalamin (B_{12}). Older people in particular are often deficient in this vitamin because their bodies simply don't absorb it easily from food. One study found that giving patients with Alzheimer's disease vitamin B_{12} along with bright-light therapy, improved their circadian rhythms and their cognitive state. In another published case report, researchers described a man who'd had trouble falling asleep and staying asleep for ten years. He finally got a good night's sleep after taking B_{12} supplements. Although researchers aren't exactly sure how B_{12} works to enhance sleep, they suspect the brain needs it to make melatonin, since supplementing appears to modulate melatonin secretion, enhance light-sensitivity, normalize circadian rhythms, and normalize the sleep/wake rhythm.

Good food sources: Meat, seafood, and dairy products. Breakfast cereals and soy products are often fortified with B_{12}.

Folic acid. This B vitamin is very helpful in treating restless legs syndrome, a condition in which uncontrollable leg movements result in insomnia. The condition is particularly prevalent in older people and pregnant women, who, studies find, generally have low iron and folate levels. For more information on restless legs syndrome, see Chapter 5.

> **Good food sources:** Liver, brewer's yeast, dark green leafy vegetables, dried beans.

Pantothenic acid. Deficiencies in this vitamin may also cause sleep problems.

> **Good food sources.** Brewer's yeast, liver, eggs, wheat germ and bran, peanuts, peas, and meats.

Copper and Iron

Studies find that deficiencies of these two trace minerals can affect your sleep. Yet Americans generally only get half the amount of dietary copper considered adequate through food, with just one in four getting the full RDA of 2 milligrams. As for iron, most Americans receive just over half the RDA (18 milligrams), while many premenopausal women are at risk of iron deficiency.

In one study, in which women were given just one-third the RDA of copper, they took 10 percent longer to fall asleep, and, while they slept longer, they awoke feeling less rested than when they received the full RDA of copper. Conversely, in a group of women receiving one-third the RDA of iron, the women slept longer than normal but woke in the middle of the night 20 percent more often than when they received the full amount.

Since only about 10 percent of dietary iron is actually absorbed, to get the 2 milligrams of absorbed iron women need and 1 milligram of absorbed iron men need, experts say you have to consume 10 to 20 milligrams daily. While food sources are your best bets, they say you can supplement these minerals as part of a comprehensive multivitamin/mineral supplement.

Good food sources: Lobster and cooked oysters are the best.

The Carbohydrate/Tryptophan Connection

You read in Chapter 2 about the effects the hormones serotonin and melatonin have on sleep. While food doesn't contain serotonin (although a few foods do contain small amounts of melatonin), some foods do contain large amounts of the precursors to these important neurotransmitters, which are then converted into serotonin and melatonin. One of these precursors is the amino acid tryptophan. You're familiar with the effects of this amino acid if you've ever wondered why you lie around in a daze after stuffing yourself with Thanksgiving turkey. Turkey is packed with tryptophan. In fact, all animal protein, including dairy products, eggs, meat, and fish, contain tryptophan.

But eating just the turkey—or any other protein source—isn't going to help your serotonin levels. That's because, like a blocked tunnel, other amino acids prevent tryptophan's passage into the brain. One way around this roadblock is to pair small amounts of protein with larger amounts of carbohydrates, effectively "unclogging" that blocked tunnel to the brain, letting the tryptophan in and enabling it to be converted to serotonin.

Sleep-Enhancing Foods

- Turkey, eggs, fish, dairy products, bananas, pineapples, spinach, whole wheat toast, and walnuts. All are good sources of tryptophan.
- A glass of warm milk with honey. This age-old sleep remedy now has some science behind it. The milk provides some protein, while the honey is pure carbohydrate.
- Baked (not fried) chips, lightly salted pretzels, graham crackers, plain or lightly salted popcorn, and fresh fruit. All can not only boost levels of serotonin through the tryptophan conversion, but can boost existing levels of serotonin as well.
- Oats, sweet corn, rice, ginger, tomatoes, bananas, and barley. All are good sources of melatonin.

Presleep Eating

Now that you know some of the foods that enhance sleep, we're going to discuss the best times to eat them.

Biggest, big, small. That's the order your meals should take. Have your largest meals (i.e., highest calories) earlier in the day, saving your smallest meal for dinner. This limits the amount of work your gastrointestinal system needs to do to digest dinner, reducing the excitatory chemicals your brain releases during this process, chemicals that keep you awake.

Keep it light. My husband and I love to eat out at fancy restaurants. Unfortunately, by the time we finish a three-hour dinner, take the babysitter home, and let the dog out, we're less than an hour from our last bite but too sleepy to keep our eyes open. Yet trying to sleep on a full stomach is like trying to sleep on a bed of nails. A better plan if you know you're going to going to sleep soon after eating out is to eat light. Skip dessert and appetizer, and have a broth-based soup and salad for dinner, or a lean piece of chicken or fish along with steamed vegetables. Come midnight when you're snoozing away instead of counting chefs, you'll be glad you did.

Find the right mix. While what you eat at breakfast isn't going to affect your night's sleep, what you eat at dinner— even an early dinner—might. That's why it's important to follow many of the Eat to Sleep tips covered in today's program, including limiting spicy, fatty foods, and building your meal around small amounts of low-fat protein coupled with larger amounts of complex carbohydrates. So tonight, fix a stir-fry with boneless chicken breast and a variety of vegetables, served over brown rice. Or broil a 3-ounce piece of salmon with a side of lentils and a large salad.

Presleep snacking. In checking over her presleep routine, Karen, 46, of Bangor, Maine, noticed one item that worried her. Every night before she went to bed, she raided the refrigerator, chowing down on leftovers from dinner, or digging into an oversized bowl of Haagen Daz. What she didn't realize was that this pattern was partly responsible for her insomnia. That's not to say she shouldn't have a presleep snack. She just needs to choose the right foods at the right time.

> **Best time:** About an hour before bed.
> **Best snack:** A little bit of protein, like a hard-boiled egg, coupled with complex carbohydrates (like a corn tortilla or whole wheat toast). The proverbial glass of warm milk will also work if it's downed with some carbohydrates, like graham crackers, because milk contains high levels of tryptophan. Milk also contains casomorphins, a

natural opiate. Or try a banana milkshake, which contains tryptophan, calcium, and vitamin B_6. Put 1 banana and 1 cup of vanilla ice cream, along with a dash of cinnamon, in the blender. Blend until it reaches milkshake consistency. Other options: Whole grain cereal with milk, yogurt with a piece of fruit, a cheese stick with a few low-sodium crackers. Or try some oatmeal. Oats are an herbal remedy often used to soothe the nerves. And, of course, oatmeal (especially drizzled with honey) is the quintessential comfort food.

Other good bedtime snacks: One slice of turkey, bananas, figs, dates, yogurt, tuna, and whole grain crackers or nut butter. All are high in tryptophan.

Night-Eating Syndrome

With this condition, people eat very little during the day, but binge late at night, then have problems falling asleep, and often wake up several times during the night and eat again. In fact, some take in half or more of their daily calories at night. This disorder affects about 1.5 percent of the general population, but as many as 10 percent of obese people who seek treatment. This disorder is likely related to disruptions in hormones and circadian rhythms, particularly melatonin and leptin (a hormone that controls appetite). People with the disorder also have elevated levels of cortisol (the stress hormone).

Researchers suspect that night eating, which consists mainly of carbohydrate snacks high in serotonin, is a way of self-medicating for underlying stress.

Sleep-Stealing Foods

Avoid overstimulating food too close to bedtime. Tacos or super-spicy Thai takeout is going to be with you as soon as you lie down, in the form of reflux, a fancy name for heartburn, in which the acids from your stomach back up into your esophagus, giving you a burning feeling or making you cough.

Also avoid:

Fruit juice. One study found that, compared to water, it took participants an extra 20 to 30 minutes before they felt drowsy after drinking fruit juice compared to how they felt after drinking water. This was probably due to the high sugar content in fruit juice.

Fatty, spicy, gas-inducing foods. Pass on the shrimp scampi (too much garlic), say no to the Texas chili (the beans and spiciness pose a double whammy), and avoid the multitude of fried appetizers (cheese, chicken, vegetables) that fill restaurant menus these days.

Tyrosine-containing foods. Tyrosine is an amino acid that increases the release of norepinephrine, a brain stimulant. It's found in bacon and other processed meats, aged cheeses like Stilton, blue, and Parmesan, and soft cheeses, like mozzarella, Swiss, Gruyere, and feta. It's also found in chocolate (which you were avoiding anyway because of its caffeine content), potatoes, sauerkraut, sugar, spinach, tomatoes, wine, and yogurt. Avoid these foods within three hours of bedtime. Ironically, milk is also full of tyrosine, but its excitatory effects are probably canceled out by the relaxing effects of the tryptophan. Milk also contains calcium, which, as noted above, is a natural relaxant. That's why you need to experiment with various foods, adding and subtracting foods on a regular basis, to determine what works best for you.

Protein. While it is a good idea to get a little bit of protein before bed (to keep blood sugar levels steady through the night and get a bit of tryptophan), more is definitely *not* better. Too much protein overstimulates your brain by causing the release of dopamine and epinephrine (adrenaline), classic "wake me up" neurotransmitters.

Avoid Aluminum

In one USDA study, researchers compared how well women who got over 1,000 milligrams of aluminum a day slept, compared to those who got just 300 milligrams. Those who got more aluminum slept worse. The major sources of aluminum are antacids, which may contain as much as 200 to 250 milligrams of aluminum per teaspoon. So chart your antacid intake for a few days in your sleep diary to see if this might be contributing to your sleep problems.

The Alcohol Dilemma

About 30 percent of people with persistent insomnia say they used alcohol in the past year to help them sleep, with 67 percent saying alcohol helped them sleep. Alcohol is, primarily, a sedative. So of course, after a bottle of wine or a few beers, you may fall asleep the instant your head hits the pillow. But then, a few hours later, once your body has metabolized the alcohol, you wake up, parched, your bladder bursting, your head aching, feeling as if there's no air in the room. You go to the bathroom, get some water, turn on the fan, then lie in bed, wide awake. This is the "rebound" effect of drinking that occurs once the alcohol is metabolized and eliminated from your body. That's because alcohol also causes the release of the stress hormone adrenaline, and blocks tryptophan from getting into your brain to form serotonin.

Even if you are one of the lucky few who don't wake up in the middle of the night after a night's drinking, chances are you'll feel terrible the next morning, with or without a hangover. Alcohol negatively affects the time you spend in the various sleep stages.

In one study, pilots drank enough alcohol between 6 p.m. and 9 p.m. to have a blood alcohol level of 0.10 and 0.12 by bedtime. The next morning, more than 14 hours after their last drink, and with a blood alcohol level of 0, they still didn't perform as well in flight simulator tests as they'd done without drinking anything the night before.

You probably don't have to pilot a plane after a few too many drinks, but you do have to drive a car and work all day. That isn't to say you shouldn't drink at all. Some studies find that, in nonalcoholics who occasionally use alcohol, light drinking (one to two drinks a day) can improve sleep. But you can develop a tolerance to these effects within three nights, and then may experience insomnia when you don't use it, a condition called alcohol-dependent sleep disorder.

Limit Caffeine

For centuries, caffeinated drinks have played a role in society. The English tradition of "afternoon tea" is scheduled at an ideal time to beat back the midafternoon doldrums. And in the 16th century, Turkish women could divorce their husbands if the man failed to keep his family's pot filled with coffee.

But Americans have taken to the fragrant bean in a big way, consuming more coffee per person than citizens of any other country. The current craze for coffee is not new; it is just the latest in a long tradition of coffeehouses that have, for hundreds of years, nurtured the artists, writers, philosophers, and politicians who met there over strong cups of coffee to fuel their discussions.

Coffee has a number of benefits.

- It is chock full of antioxidants—substances that help repair some of the wear and tear your body experiences from the activities of daily living.
- It can perk you up in as little as 10 minutes.
- It improves safe driving by reducing reaction times.
- It improves your ability to do math.
- It lifts mild depression.
- It may protect against cavities, bladder cancer, and Parkinson's disease.

What coffee doesn't do, at least in most people, is help you fall asleep. In fact, legend has it that coffee beans were discovered when an Arabic goatherd noticed his flock became quite hyper after munching on berries from one particular bush. The reason for the energetic goats? Caffeine. One study found that a single cup of coffee drunk two hours before bed could more than double the amount of time it takes to fall asleep.

Caffeine is related to adenosine, a neurotransmitter that binds to certain receptors in brain cells, slowing down nerve cell activity and inducing drowsiness. But when you introduce caffeine into your system, the caffeine takes over those receptors, preventing adenosine from latching on. Thus, you not only don't get the relaxing effects of adenosine, but the caffeine makes those nerve cells speed up, increasing neuron firings in your brain and giving you a jolt of energy. With all this excitement going on, your pituitary gland releases hormones that tell your adrenal glands to release adrenaline, the fight-or-flight hormone.

Caffeine also lowers melatonin levels. One study found that drinking coffee at 8 p.m. lowered melatonin levels for at least six hours. And even decaffeinated coffee isn't completely free of caffeine, as the chart below shows. Additionally, some of the chemicals used to remove the caffeine in commercially prepared decaffeinated coffee can be harmful.

While its effects are felt almost immediately, caffeine also hangs around a while. About half the caffeine you consume at 7 p.m. is still in your body at 11 p.m. The older you are, the longer it remains.

Coffee is not the only caffeine-containing food/drink. There's chocolate, for instance, which, in addition to caffeine, contains the stimulant theobromine. The darker the chocolate, the higher the levels of caffeine and theobromine. Soft drinks also have extremely high levels of caffeine. Other hidden sources of caffeine include coffee ice cream (one cup of Starbucks' contains 40 to 60 milligrams of caffeine), and even coffee-flavored yogurt (45 milligrams in Dannon).

CAFFEINE LEVELS

Food/Beverage/Drug	Caffeine
Coffee (5-oz. cup)	
Brewed	60–180 mg
Instant	30–120 mg
Cappuccino (8 oz)	89 mg
Espresso (1 oz.)	89 mg
Latte (8 oz)	89 mg
Decaffeinated	5 mg

Food/Beverage/Drug	Caffeine
Tea (5-oz. cup)	
Brewed	60–180 mg
Instant	25–50 mg
Iced (12 oz)	67–76 mg
Snapple (16 oz)	48 mg
Herbal teas	0
Chocolate	
Dark chocolate (1.5 oz)	32 mg
Milk chocolate (1.5 oz)	9 mg
Hot cocoa (5 oz)	15 mg
Soft drinks (12 oz)	
Coke or Pepsi	37 mg
Tab	44 mg
Sunkist Orange	42 mg
Mountain Dew	52 mg
Sprite	0
Non-prescription drugs	
Dexatrim	200 mg
No Doz	100 mg
Excedrin (2 tablets)	65 mg
Midol (2 tablets)	64 mg
Dristan (1 tablet)	16 mg

Nocturnal Hypoglycemia

If you've ever woken up hungry in the middle of the night, you might be suffering from a mild form of nocturnal hypoglycemia. Particularly prevalent in people with diabetes, or those who have low blood sugar, or hypoglycemia, the awakening is caused when there's a drop in blood sugar. This drop, in turn, releases hormones that call upon your body to release more glucose from stored glycogen. All this action, of course, has a stimulating effect that wakes you up. You may have hypoglycemia without even knowing it. One government study found that almost half of all Americans experience hypoglycemia at some time or other.

To avoid this middle-of-the-night activity, make sure your presleep snack contains a bit of protein (which takes longer to digest and maintains more even blood sugar levels) and complex carbohydrates, such as whole grain bread or crackers, instead of simple carbohydrates, such as sugar, foods made with white flour, or alcohol. If you do wake up hungry in the middle of the night, try not to eat anything. By eating, you're simply rewarding yourself for the midnight awakening, which could quickly become a bad habit.

If you think you suffer from hypoglycemia—you wake up in the middle of the night hungry, have dramatic mood swings depending on when you last ate, and crave sweets—ask your doctor for a blood test.

Quit Smoking

If a cigarette is the first thing you reach for in the morning and the last thing you reach for at night, smoking may be the reason you're having trouble sleeping. Nicotine—the active ingredient in tobacco—is a well-known stimulant. Because nicotine is absorbed through the mucous membranes in your mouth, it gets to your brain quickly, producing a feeling of alert calm. Nicotine is also addictive, with cravings for the next smoke beginning about an hour after you finish the first.

Smoking interferes with sleep on two levels: Its stimulative effects prevent you from falling asleep, and its addictive nature can trigger cravings strong enough to wake you up in the middle of the night. Studies of smokers who go through at least one pack a day find that they take longer to fall asleep and they don't sleep as well once they are asleep.

Other effects of smoking on sleep:

- Its effects on your respiratory system often lead to a chronic cough and mucus buildup, which can interfere with a good night's sleep.
- By reducing your ability to take in oxygen, it can cause you to have several mini-awakenings each night, just as you would with sleep apnea. While you aren't aware of the awakenings, the disrupted sleep leaves you feeling exhausted the next day.

The Program: Day 4

Today you're going to eat a healthy diet filled with whole grains and low-fat protein by following the Meal Plan below. You're also going to:

- Stop with one cup of coffee or tea in the morning.
- Give up your 4 p.m. chocolate bar in favor of a handful of nuts or a carton of non-fat yogurt.
- Serve dinner at 6 p.m. instead of 8 p.m.
- Water down your wine with seltzer water to make a wine spritzer—and reduce your alcohol intake.
- Avoid using any antacids, especially a liquid antacid.
- Take a balanced multivitamin/mineral supplement in the morning.
- Take a calcium/magnesium supplement in the evening 30 minutes before bedtime.

A Beginning Meal Plan

Breakfast
Whole grain toast spread with peanut butter
1 cup orange juice
1 pear
1 cup coffee or tea (preferably decaffeinated)

Lunch
2 pieces whole wheat bread spread with 1 cup tuna
   salad (water-packed tuna mixed with 1 tablespoon
   low-fat mayonnaise, shredded carrots, and minced
   onion
2 cups green salad with 2 tablespoons low-fat Italian
   dressing and cup ¼ garbanzo beans mixed in
1 cup cut-up fruit
1 cup skim milk or diluted apple juice

Dinner (eaten at least 3 hours before you go to bed)
3 ounces broiled fish
1 cup steamed green beans
Tossed salad with low-fat dressing on the side
1 cup quinoa
1 cup grapes
1 cup skim milk

Snack (1 hour before bed)
Cereal with skim milk, *or*
1 cup skim milk with 2 graham crackers, *or*
1 ounce turkey with 1 ounce cheese and 3 whole
   wheat crackers

Tomorrow: Exercise your way to sleep.

DAY 5: EXERCISE TO SLEEP

"Despite frequent advice from experts telling people not to exercise vigorously before sleep, I do. Most nights I do about 10 to 15 miles on an exercycle between 9 and 11 p.m. before bed. If I don't exercise, all my daytime anxieties build up and I never get to sleep. I consider this an essential detox experience. During the summer months, my husband and I take an after-dinner walk. That knocks him out. While it relaxes me, I still need the mind-numbing effect of the exercycle."
—Bev Bennett, Evanston, Il.

"Swimming is the absolute best thing for a good night's sleep. I don't know why. I think it's because swimming relaxes you so completely (mind, body, and muscles) and it's a great workout. I always sleep well after I go swimming."
—Mary Beth, Savannah, Ga.

I hate to exercise. Yet every time I go out for a brisk walk, force myself to do 20 minutes on the stationary bike in our basement, or lift a few weights, I feel better, both emotionally and physically. Exercise causes the brain to release feel-good hormones called endorphins. But it does much more than that when it comes to its ability to affect your sleep:

- By exposing you to sunlight and fresh air (if you exercise outside), it helps balance your circadian rhythms, or sleep/wake cycle.
- By helping you maintain a healthy weight, exercise reduces the risk of sleep disorders such as sleep apnea.
- By working out your muscles, exercise leaves you with relaxed muscles when it's time for bed.
- By providing a release button for nervous energy and stress, exercise puts you in a more peaceful

state of mind when it's time to turn the lights out. It also helps release the lactic acid that tends to build up with stress. In fact, the American Council on Exercise (ACE) notes that one exercise session generates 90 to 120 minutes of "relaxation response."

Consistent exercise also increases levels of hormones that contribute to sleep and calm, including serotonin, dopamine, and acetylcholine. These hormones help you relax by keeping your heart rate and blood pressure low.

The regular increase and then fall in temperature that exercise creates helps with melatonin release and sleep readiness in much the same way a hot bath helps your temperature rise and then fall. This drop in body temperature persists as long as four hours after exercise.

Studies find that insomniacs tend to lead more sedentary lives than people who have no problems falling and staying asleep. There's even some evidence that exercise can help with another sleep-stealing disorder, restless legs syndrome (see Chapter 5).

Personal trainer Selene Yeager, author of the book *Perfectly Fit* (Rodale, 2001), says 75 percent of her clients tell her that they sleep most soundly when they're participating in a regular exercise program of at least 30 minutes of moderate to vigorous exercise most days of the week, including jogging, swimming, cycling, brisk walking, and/or strength training. "One client owns his own business and has a good bit of stress," says Yeager. "In the five years I've been working with him, he tells me that whenever he misses a day or two, he ends up lying in bed wide-eyed because he can't shut down.'"

Exercise promotes relaxation in so many ways, Yeager says. "Maybe most importantly, it improves our body's ability to manage stress, and that increased stress resistance means less time staring at the numbers on the clock, worrying about your next project or your son who has just started driving." Exercise also helps blow off any present stress you're struggling with, she says, which is why many people find exercising after work ideal.

Yet less than 10 percent of Americans exercise four times a week. In one survey of 2,002 people, nearly one in four said that nothing—not their doctor's advice, pleading from their family, or access to workout facilities—would increase their physical activity.

While none of those things may turn you toward an exercise routine either, maybe the promise of a good night's sleep will. Consider that in a 2001 *Consumer Reports* survey of 46,000 people, respondents said exercise was almost as effective—and sometimes more effective—than medications for common medical problems including insomnia. Forty-six thousand people can't all be wrong.

Exercise and Sleep: The Scientific Evidence

Sleep researchers just love studying people and their sleep habits. What's really amazing are all the people willing to be kept up at odd hours, or to sleep with electrodes attached to their head and body, or to spend days, even weeks, isolated in sleep labs. But the results are worth it, especially when it comes to the effects of exercise on sleep. Consider the evidence.

In one study, about 300 men and 400 women all reduced their sleep disorders by engaging in regular activity at least once a week, participating regularly in an exercise program, and walking at a normal pace for more than six blocks a day.

In another study, Stanford University researchers had a group of 43 people with mild sleep problems, who lived fairly sedentary lives, exercise four times a week. Twice a week they participated in an organized aerobics class, including 30 minutes of endurance training. The other two times they exercised on their own for 40 minutes, walking briskly or riding a stationary bike. After 16 weeks in this program, they were able to fall asleep 15 minutes earlier, and sleep about 45 minutes longer at night.

Studies find that mild to moderate exercise can even improve symptoms of sleep apnea, leading to fewer incidences of interrupted breathing, and thus an overall better night's sleep.

In a 10-week study of 32 volunteers aged 60 and older, one-third of those who exercised their leg, hip, and upper torso muscles on pneumatic resistance equipment for 45 minutes, three times each week, improved their sleep quality, while nearly all improved in terms of depression. A control group, which attended a health education meeting, had no such improvements.

Review and Reflect

Look back over your sleep diary, and note the days that you were more physically active. Did you sleep better those nights? The proof of the benefits of exercise on sleep should act as motivation to get you moving.

Exercise Defined

Exercise is, simply, movement. The Surgeon General recommends we get 30 minutes on most or all days of the week. Those 30 minutes don't have to occur all at once, and they don't have to occur as part of "typical" exercise. You might already be getting this 30 minutes without even knowing it just participating in your normal activities. All you may need to do is increase the time you spend on particular activities. For instance, 30 minutes of the following activities burns as many or more calories (for a 150-pound woman) as a brisk walk (which burns 136 calories):

Shoveling snow	204 calories
Outside carpentry	204 calories
Scrubbing the floor or mowing the lawn (with a push mower):	187 calories
Fast dancing	187 calories
Gardening	170 calories

Even simple changes in your everyday activities can make a difference:

- Park at the farthest edge of the parking lot wherever you go.
- Take the stairs if you're going ten floors or less.
- Instead of sending an office E-mail message, get up and walk over to your colleague's desk to deliver the message.
- Hide all remote controls.
- Make drive-throughs off-limits. Even parking your car, or walking to the restaurant or bank or dry cleaner, gets you moving.
- Get a dog. This works particularly well if you don't have a yard. You can't just let the dog out, but must walk it.
- If you take public transportation to work, get off a stop or two before your usual one and walk the rest of the way.
- Instead of having lunch or coffee with a friend, go for a walk.
- Institute walking business meetings for one-on-one meetings.

Getting Started

Consider Your Physical Condition

The American Council on Exercise (ACE) recommends you ask yourself the following questions before beginning any exercise program:

1. Have you been told you have a heart condition and should only participate in physical activity recommended by a doctor?
2. Do you feel pain (or discomfort) in your chest when you do physical activity? When you are not participating in physical activity? While at rest, do you frequently experience fast, irregular heartbeats or very slow beats?
3. Do you ever become dizzy and lose your balance, or lose consciousness? Have you fallen more than twice in the past year (no matter what the reason)?
4. Do you have a bone or joint problem that could worsen as a result of physical activity? Do you have pain in your legs or buttocks when you walk?
5. Do you take blood pressure or heart medications?
6. Do you have any cuts or wounds on your feet that don't seem to heal?
7. Have you experienced unexplained weight loss in the past six months?
8. Are you aware of any reason why you should not participate in physical activity?

If you answered "no" to all of these questions, then you have passed the first round of questions, and you can be reasonably sure that you can safely take part in at least a moderate physical activity program. But if you are a man over 40 or a woman over 50 and want to exercise more vigorously, check with your physician before starting. And if you answered yes to any of the questions, see a doctor before you start exercising, regardless of your age.

Start Slow

Begin to exercise slowing, gradually building up to the point where you are working at 55 to 80 percent of your estimated maximum target heart rate (220 minus your age). To measure your heart rate, take your pulse as soon as you stop exercising. Count your heartbeat for ten seconds, then multiply that by six to convert it to a one-minute heart rate. So, if your heart beats 24 times in 10 seconds, your one-minute heart rate would be 144. If you're 35, your target heart rate is 185. Eighty percent of 185 equals 148. That's the highest your heart rate should be while exercising.

Stretch

Before you begin your workout, warm and prepare your muscles with light stretching, generally about five to ten minutes, to avoid injury.

Pace Yourself

The adage "no pain, no gain" is just plain wrong. Exercise experts recommend that you work out at a comfortable pace, never working so hard that you can't carry on a conversation, or that you're above your target heart rate.

Schedule It

Three to four days of aerobic activity a week should help with your sleep problems. If you're looking to lose weight, aim for four or more days a week. Always take at least one day off a week.

Time It

Work up to 20 or more minutes per session as part of your Seven-Day Sleep Program.

When to Exercise

Most articles or books on exercise and sleep recommend that you not exercise within two to three hours of bedtime. Exercise raises your body temperature, and, as we've already learned, your temperature needs to drop slightly to increase melatonin levels and ready your body for sleep. But a 1999 study questions that assumption. Researchers at the University of California at San Diego examined the effect of intense, prolonged exercise just before sleep in 16 competitive male cyclists. On the experimental night, the men either exercised under bright light for three hours, or sat under bright light for three hours, beginning 90 minutes before their usual bedtime, then went to bed a half hour afterward. The researchers found no difference in either group's ability to sleep.

One caveat: The physical fitness of the volunteers may have played a role in their ability to exercise so soon before sleep and still fall asleep. The take-home message: The better shape you're in, the more likely it is that you'll be able to exercise just before bed and still get a good night's sleep.

Still, most sleep experts recommend exercise four to five hours before bedtime.

I think what's most important is that you exercise at all . . . regardless of the time of day. So this is another item to track in your sleep diary over the next two weeks: Vary your exercise routine from early morning to midday to just before dinner to about two hours before you go to sleep. Compare when you exercised to how you slept, and see if any patterns emerge.

Finding the Right Exercise for You

To figure out what works best to get you moving, think about things you most enjoy. Do you love watching your kids play soccer? Then look into an adult soccer league in your area. Do you enjoy nature? Call your local parks department and get a list of walking/hiking trails in your area.

While it's true that aerobic exercise seems to provide the greatest benefits in terms of sleep, that could also be because there's been very little research looking at non-aerobic workouts like yoga in terms of sleep.

Think about where to exercise. Although 33 million Americans belong to a health club, there are pros and cons of joining a club. For instance, on the pro side, a health club has top-of-the-line, well-maintained equipment and trained staff on hand to help you use it, as well as regularly scheduled classes. But you have to make sure you have the time to get to the health club, and the cost may be a deterrent. Still, clubs are generally open long hours, and provide a safe, climate-controlled environment for working out— even when it's raining outside.

Other tips to get you moving:

Feed your mind. Check out books-on-tape from the library and listen to them as you walk. You'll get so wrapped up in the story you probably won't mind going the extra mile.

Go in style. Sometimes the right equipment can make all the difference. Invest in some quality walking (or running) shoes, a reflective vest (for nighttime and early morning walks/runs), and some stylish exercise clothing.

Buy some toys. Exercise balls, resistance bands, neon-colored hand weights, yoga mats, and chinning bars can all add an element of "play" to your workout.

Reinvent old joys. Did you used to play tennis? Then take it up again. Treat yourself to lessons. Enjoy golf? Walking an 18-hole course is great exercise. Love to dance? Ballroom classes are a fabulous way to get in your 30 minutes and spend some valuable time with your partner (or meet someone new, if you're single).

Break it up. Remember that these 30 minutes can occur any time of the day. So, if you take your dog on three 10-minute walks a day, you've met your requirement.

Consider new methods. Low-impact exercise programs like yoga, Pilates and tai chi can provide excellent strength training as well as aerobic workouts that leave you more relaxed and flexible.

The Program: Day 5

As we noted earlier, one day of exercise isn't necessarily going to resolve your sleep problems. You need to commit to increasing your physical activity at least four days a week. But you have to start somewhere, and today is the day. Follow the easy Exercise Plan below for now; you can develop your own personalized plan as time goes on.

A Beginning Exercise Plan

In the morning. Before you get into your shower, spend 15 minutes doing some light stretching and calisthenics.

During the day. Find any excuse you can to move. Follow some of the tips listed earlier. If you can, get out for a walk during lunch. Even walking up and down the stairs in your building counts. Keep your tennis shoes, socks, and an extra set of clothes with some deodorant in your car or office. You'll never have an excuse not to take a brisk 10-minute walk. Fit in some regular exercise, such as brisk walking, spinning class, lap swimming, a game of tennis—whatever you like—at least 30 minutes a day most days of the week.

Just before bed. From personal trainer Selene Yeager comes a simple bedtime workout that can benefit everyone from beginning exercisers to seasoned athletes. The idea behind this yoga-inspired routine is to stretch and release the tension in your major muscles. By making this part of your nightly winding-down ritual, you relax your body and your mind. As a bonus, performing this routine nightly will increase your flexibility, which improves your posture and your performance in other exercise.

Hold each pose for 20 seconds, breathing deeply and clearing your mind as you stretch. Go through the routine two to three times. For best results, wear loose clothing you can move freely in, and dim the lights. When you get the hang of the moves, they'll flow gracefully into one another.

Standing Arch: Stand with your feet slightly apart, arms down at your sides. Then sweep your arms out in front of you, lifting them overhead, while arching your head up and back slightly to look toward the ceiling. Place your palms together for a deeper stretch. Hold, while breathing deeply. Release.

Standing Fold: Stand with your feet slightly apart. Sweep your arms out to the side, while slowly bending forward from the hips. Bring your fingertips to the floor (or as far down as you can) just in front of your toes, bending your knees if you need to. Hold, while breathing deeply. Release.

Cat and Cow: Position yourself on your hands and knees. Round your back up toward the ceiling while you drop your head toward the floor. Hold, while breathing into the stretch. Release, then immediately drop your navel toward the floor, arching your back, while you lift your head and look up toward the ceiling. Hold, while breathing into the stretch. Release.

Child's Pose: Kneel with the top of your feet on the floor, toes pointed behind you. Sit back onto your heels and bend forward from the hips, lowering your torso to your thighs. Stretch your arms overhead and rest your palms and forehead on the floor (or as close to it as comfortably possible). Hold, while breathing into the stretch. Release.

———

Tomorrow we'll explore finding your way to a good night's sleep when you sleep with someone.

DAY 6: SLEEPING WITH SOMEONE

"Most people who sleep normally don't understand us light sleepers. They don't understand why we would rather spend $150 on a hotel room rather than sleep on the floor of their apartment, for example. I was once in a very awkward position when someone asked to room with me at a conference to save money. I said no. If I room with someone I don't know well, my sleep is gone."

—Alisa Bauman, Emmaus, Pa.

I love my husband. But I relish the nights when he's traveling, because then I know I'll get a good night's sleep. No lying awake listening to him snore. No waking up in the middle of the night because he's snoring. No kicking him in the shins, hitting his back, threatening to sleep in the other room because he's snoring.

As you can see, my husband's snoring disrupts my ability to fall asleep and stay asleep. But I'm not alone. One study found that 86 percent of women surveyed said their husbands snored, and over half said their sleep was disrupted by it. Of the men surveyed, just 57 percent said their wives snored, and only 15 percent said they were bothered by it.

But snoring isn't the only problem. You may like the room hot and your partner likes it cold. Or you prefer silk sheets and your partner wants flannel. One likes to cuddle, the other can't bear to be touched. Whatever the differences, this is called "spousal arousal syndrome." It's a serious problem, especially since couples spend nearly one-third of their lives together sleeping. No wonder a 1994 British study found that couples who are used to sharing a bed actually sleep longer and better when they sleep alone.

Bottom line: The person or pet who shares your bed may

be the reason for your own sleep problems. Today's program addresses this problem.

The Cacophony of Snoring

With habitual snoring common in at least 44 percent of men and 28 percent of women, it's safe to assume there are a number of people lying awake at night. Rumor has it that a Texas gunfighter named John Wesley Hardin once fired a shot at another snorer in the next room, killing him. And it could explain National Sleep Foundation findings that more than one in ten married adults (12 percent) report sleeping alone.

As the father of all sleep research, William Dement, wrote in an editorial in the October 1999, *Mayo Clinic Proceedings:* "We should . . . keep at the front of our minds that for every snoring patient we evaluate and treat, we are improving the lives of two people."

No wonder that when Mayo Clinic researchers studied ten married couples in which the husband was being evaluated for snoring and obstructive sleep apnea, they found that once the man's snoring was treated with a device similar to an oxygen mask, the women got an extra hour of sleep a night.

Anatomy of a Snore

When you snore, your soft palate and uvula, the fleshy tip that hangs down in the back of your throat, vibrate. The vibration is usually caused by turbulent airflow moving through your mouth or nose. Turbulent airflow can also come from the base of your tongue or from some parts of your throat. The same physical phenomenon that causes your shower curtain to be sucked toward the shower water when you turn the shower on, called the Bernoulli effect, is what causes the snoring sound. For, as any physics student could tell you, any fast flow of air will try to lift and vibrate those things the air passes by. It's the irregularity of that airflow—the fact that it's not smooth—that causes the alternating vibration of the soft palate.

A Shot for Snoring

A new treatment for snoring, called injection snoreplasty, is cheap (about $35), relatively painless, and can be performed in 15 minutes in a doctor's office. It works like this: Your soft palate (the soft, upper part of your mouth near the back of your throat), is numbed with a topical anesthetic, and then sodium tetradecyl sulfate, which stiffens the palate with scar tissue, is injected. About two minutes later, the injected area turns purple as the drug takes effect. The procedure is still new and no long-term effects are known, yet studies find that even after a year, 92 percent of patients say their snoring is gone or is no longer a problem. Before talking to your physician about this procedure, however, make sure he/she rules out sleep apnea as a cause of your snoring. For more on sleep apnea, see page 147.

Beyond Snoring

Snoring is not the only reason sleeping with someone else can disrupt your sleep. Consider sleeping patterns. For instance, I tend to stay up late working, while my husband, who has to get up at 5:30 a.m. to make a grueling commute, is usually asleep by 10 p.m. When I do crawl into bed, he's snoring away, and all I can do is lie there in the dark. In other relationships, things are flipped. A light sleeper who goes to bed first could be awakened by the sounds of his partner washing up and climbing into bed.

Even your partner's state of mind can affect your sleep.

If you both go to bed at the same time, but she's stressed and anxious, tossing and turning with her own insomnia, that could be enough to keep you awake, even though you've been following all the steps outlined for the previous five days of the Seven-Day Sleep Program.

Simply having another person in bed with you is enough to disrupt your sleep. One study found that half of all movements by one sleeper trigger movements by the other within 30 seconds. (An average adult sleeper changes positions between 20 and 60 times a night.) Men seem to be more restless than women. Maybe this doesn't sound like much of a problem, but the reality is that any motion transferred across the surface of a mattress—as when he rolls over or she turns on her side and kicks out her leg—can affect your depth of sleep, thus making you more vulnerable to waking up at the slightest noise and pulling you out of the restorative deep sleep stage.

Review and Reflect

Flip through your sleep diary. Note who was in your bed each night (include your pets) and how you ranked your night's sleep. Did you go to bed first or did your partner? Did you fall asleep quickly but then wake up due to snoring or movement? Did you wake up too early because your partner woke before you? Identify any patterns. This will help you know which steps below to concentrate on.

Examine the Setting

You learned on the first day of the Seven-Day Sleep Program about the importance of the right setting for sleep, including the proper mattress and the correct colors and decor for your bedroom. Now review your bedroom with an eye toward your sleeping partner.

How big is your bed? If you usually sleep with someone, is your bed big enough? Many people swear by a king-sized bed, which provides room enough for partners, children, and pets. Can't get a king-sized into your room? Try pushing two full-sized beds together, or, if you need even more space, consider a queen-sized and a single. For tonight, how about moving the twin bed from the guest room into your bedroom to make your bed larger. If you have time, stop by a department or linen store for one of the kits available to connect twin beds into one seamless, king-sized bed.

Remake your bed. Put a separate blanket and top sheet on each side, so you don't have to worry about your partner hogging the blankets. If you prefer satin and he likes cotton, make up the bed with separate sheets.

Adjust the temperature. Does the room always feel too warm to you and too cool to your him/her? Buy your partner an electric blanket today, then tonight, open the window just a crack or turn down the heat. Search for a compromise.

Raise the head of your bed. Snoring and sleep apnea only get worse with nasal congestion. Raising your partner's head will help those passages drain. Place several wooden blocks, bricks, or even heavy books under the legs at the head of the bed before you get into bed tonight. That will raise your partner's head (and yours), enhancing nasal drainage and reducing storing.

Prepare your sleeping partner

You can't stop your partner from moving in his or her sleep, but there are numerous things you can do to help reduce your partner's snoring.

Start with dinner. Make it light, and alcohol free. Alcohol relaxes throat muscles that vibrate, leading to snoring. And digesting a heavy meal is a sure way to ensure a restless evening. Fat and animal protein also increase muscle relaxation, which causes that pharyngeal tissue in the back of the throat to relax, resulting in snoring.

Second, keep your partner away from ice cream and cookies after dinner. Instead, prepare a snack of sleep-inducing food, such as graham crackers and warm milk, as described in Day 4 of the program, to relax both of you before sleep. Continue with this regimen for several weeks, and the snoring may decline or disappear altogether, since weight is a contributing factor to snoring.

Hide the cigarettes. Cigarettes irritate and inflame the upper airways and throat tissue, narrowing them and making them more likely to vibrate.

Get a tennis ball. Sew a pocket into the back of your partner's pajama top or T-shirt and stuff it with the ball. This will keep your partner from rolling onto his/her back and snoring. Sleeping on the back pulls the tongue farther back into the mouth, causing it to vibrate with each inhalation, resulting in a snuffling snore.

Buy some Breathe Rights. Breathe Rights are over-the-counter nose splints that open the nostrils wider, improving breathing and decreasing snoring. A Swedish study of 35 habitual snorers and their partners found Breathe Rights significantly reduced snoring. Present them gift-wrapped to your partner during dinner.

Try a nasal spray. If your partner is congested, suggest a decongestant before bedtime that opens and unclogs nasal passages. Have your partner immerse his/her nose in a cup of warm salt water, inhale through the nose until he/she feels the water in the back of the throat, then blow the nose, ejecting the salt water. Repeat two or three times. This clears the nasal passages.

Try a massage. A massage or a hot bath or shower is particularly helpful if your partner is anxious or stressed and his/her tossing and turning is keeping you awake.

Make love. It can relax your partner (and you) enough so that dropping off to sleep quickly—and staying asleep—is a given.

Prepare Yourself

Buy some earplugs. And use them!

Go to bed first. That way, by the time your partner gets into bed, you'll already be asleep, and you'll be less likely to lie awake hearing the snoring.

Try soft music. When her snoring kept her husband, Vance, lying awake nights, Catherine Grozier of Bethlehem, Pennsylvania, bought him a bedside CD player with headphones. These days, he puts a soothing, new age CD into the player, slips the headphones over his ears, and drifts off to sleep with no problem.

What About the Kids?

"I sleep with my six-year-old son. Some folks would say that's weird. I started when he was much younger and was scared to sleep alone, it just got us more sleep so that when he woke up in the middle of the night, he didn't scream and cry and come into our room saying he was scared. Now

he's not really scared so much as I like sleeping in his room, on his mattress, and snuggling with my baby boy while he's still little. Also, after he falls asleep, I can turn on the reading light and do crosswords . . . whereas I can't do that with my husband. I know our society would frown on our practice, but this works well for my family and my son is growing up happy, healthy, and feeling quite loved and secure."
   —Judy, New York City

If you have children who crawl into bed with you, a good night's sleep can be hard to find. Married people with children average less sleep during the week than those without children (6.7 vs. 7.2 hours a night), and single people without children (7.1 hours). More than one in ten married adults (12 percent) with children reports typically sleeping with a child; a vast majority of those adults (81 percent) reports a sleep problem, according to the National Sleep Foundation.

Whether or not you deliberately set out to have a family bed, you may find you have one, as first one, then another, child climbs into bed with you. Approximately 30 percent of children 1 to 4 years old require a parent at least once during the night, notes sleep researcher James B. Maas in *Power Sleep* (Villard Books, 1998).

Catherine Grozier, of Bethlehem, Pennsylvania, has had at least one of her two children in bed with her and her husband every night since her oldest was born five years ago. So how does she sleep? "Well . . . I have a fitful night's sleep," she admits. Her two-year-old daughter, who generally winds up in bed with her around midnight, kicks, rubs her hair, talks in her ear, or snuggles close. Many nights the additional child sends her husband Vance, already a light sleeper, onto the basement couch in search of some rest. The lost sleep is worth it, though, Grozier says. "I just like cuddling with her."

If you're ready to reclaim your bed for your own, try these suggestions:

- **Keep a nightlight on in your child's room.** If your child awakens in the night, the dark won't terrify her.
- **Play soft sounds.** Either softly playing music on a radio or a white noise machine can help soothe your child back to sleep during nighttime awakenings.
- **Provide a "cuddly."** This could be a small stuffed animal, a blanket, even an old shirt of yours—something your child can snuggle with when she wakes up in the middle of the night.
- **Put your child back in bed.** Remind her that Mommy and Daddy sleep in their own bed, and she needs to sleep in her own bed. This may necessitate some lost sleep for you for a night or two, but the reward of having your own bed back will be worth it.
- **Don't let him/her have chocolate or soda or any other caffeine-containing food or drink before bed.** While the caffeine may not prevent her from falling asleep, it may, as we learned on Day 4 of the program, disrupt her sleep later.

Reconsider Your Pet

An estimated one in five dog and cat owners let their pet sleep on the bed with them, according to a 2002 Mayo Clinic Sleep Disorders Center study. The study found that dogs and cats are one of the biggest causes of humans' sleep problems. One patient told Center medical director John Shepard, M.D., she frequently got up in the middle of the night to let the dog out, waiting up to 15 minutes before returning to bed with her pet. He also found that 21 percent of the dogs and 7 percent of the cats snored.

It wasn't snoring that led writer Alisa Bauman to kick her 63-pound Doberman, Rhodes, out of her bed. She and her husband allowed Rhodes to burrow under the covers with them. "But after about two hours, he'd get too hot, stand up, pulling the covers off, shake off the covers, jump onto the floor, shake his head back and forth (which makes his ears flop loudly from side to side), and then lie on the floor to cool down." Then, an hour later, instead of jumping back into the bed, he'd sit on the floor and whine until either Alisa or her husband let him back into bed.

"I decided that he could no longer be under the covers with us," she said. Easier said than done. To keep him from constantly pressing his nose at the top of the covers to try to root his way under, she gave him his own blanket and made him lie down in the middle of the bed toward her feet (where he can't take up too much space) and covered him with the blanket. "The best part is that he doesn't get over-heated under only one blanket, and if he does, he can kick it off without standing up and flapping his ears." She also tries to tire him out as much as possible during the day, by getting him to run, either while attached to her bike, at a dog park, or off leash while hiking, which seems to help him sleep through the night without constantly rearranging himself.

Most important, she says, "whenever the dog—or my husband's snoring—wakes me up, I've promised myself that I will move to the bedroom upstairs, where I always sleep soundly because of the lack of distractions."

Sleeping with your pet is a controversial issue, with dog trainers in particular advising against it. Beyond the issues of smell, lost sleep, and interrupted love life, there's the power issue. As a pack animal, your dog feels that claiming the obvious position of power on your bed will make her your household's dominant member. Just consider how she acts when you try to make the bed; if she's fighting you for control of the comforter, you've got a problem.

If you have a cat, take the advice of Constance Young, a writer and editor from Pine Plains, New York, who sleeps with 14 cats in her bed, at least one of which is constantly vying for the best spot. She's found it helps if she keeps the room cool and huddles under a soft comforter. "In this way, I can barely feel the cats as they dance around on the bed." The problem comes when she stays overnight in a hotel. "I feel somehow adrift without having a companion animal around, although I may sleep somewhat better on these occasions," she admits.

Deborah Mitchell uses one of her four cats as a sleep aid. "A purring cat sleeping curled up next to my stomach is calming," says the Tuscon, Arizona, writer.

If you're serious about getting a good night's sleep, you have to reconsider the pet, particularly the dog. Cats, while still a bit of a problem, tend to be smaller and less obtrusive. So tonight is the night to retake control of your bed. To do that, you first have to make sure your pet has a suitable place to sleep.

Buy your dog his/her own special bed, or move your dog's crate into your bedroom at night. That way he'll know you're nearby, and yet won't be licking your ear just as you're deep within that dream about winning the lottery. And check out the vast variety of beds out there. You can buy special heated beds, cooled beds, even wrought iron dog beds with their very own headboard. For your cat, try a special cat condo, or window seat perch, perhaps sprinkled with catnip, to keep him off your bed.

One tip: If you've let your pup sleep with you, either in bed or in your bedroom, and you want to settle him farther away, try doing it gradually. Move his bed a little farther away from you each night and train him not to jump on the bed. Many dogs will choose to sleep right outside their owner's door.

When your pet tries to reclaim his previous territory, you must be strong. Firmly put him back into his bed. It will only take a few times before he gets the message. And if you find you miss him . . . well, get a stuffed dog. At least they don't snore!

The Program: Day 6

If you sleep with someone (or something), consider all the ways it may be negatively affecting your slumber. Then work through the suggestions for improving the sleeping relationship—even if that means finding a way to sleep alone. Then spend one night sleeping apart and compare the quality of your sleep that night to when you sleep with your partner (or pet). If you find that you slept much better, but you're not ready to begin sleeping alone every night, begin working your way through the list of remedies and see which, if any, still let you get a good night's sleep with someone.

Tomorrow, we'll put together all we've learned.

They Don't Have Any Problems Sleeping!

While your dog, cat, or gerbil, or even bubbling fish may be keeping you up nights, animals themselves seem to have no sleep problems. Consider how much sleep some animals get:

	Hours per day of sleep
Donkey	3
Horse	3
Giraffe	3
Elephant	4
Goat	4
Cow	4
Dolphin	7
Rabbit	8
Guinea pig	8
Dog	9
Chimpanzee	10
Gorilla	12
Mouse	13
Hamster	14
Cat	15
Opposum	19
Bat	20

Day 7: Putting It All Together to Create Your Own Sleep Program

Congratulations! You've made it to the final day of the program. This is where it all comes together, where everything you've learned works together in lovely synchronicity to ensure you a good night's sleep.

Over and over again in the program we've told you that you need to do what works for you, regardless of what the "rules" say or even what the research shows. For just as your insomnia is unique to you, so, too, will your sleep program be unique. To get you started, however, I've put together four plans for four different types of insomnia/sleep problems. Use the one that comes closest to your own situation as a jumping-off place for custom-designing your own plan.

Each of these plans assumes that you've kept your sleep diary for at least a week.

The Lie-in-Bed-Staring-at-the-Clock Insomnia

This is the kind of insomnia most people think of when they think of insomnia.

Reevaluate your bed. (See Day 1 of the program.) How comfortable is your bed? If you don't think you need a new mattress, then at least invest in some new, ultra-comfortable sheets and a new pillow.

Orient your bedroom to sleep only. Get rid of the computer and television in your bedroom. Hide your clock so you're not staring at it. Buy blackout curtains and a white noise machine.

Prepare yourself for sleep. One hour before you want to fall asleep, get into your pajamas, turn the television off, put the bills and work away, and turn off the computer. Read a good book (not too stimulating, though), work a crossword, or put together a jigsaw puzzle.

Have a nighttime tea. Fix yourself a tea of valerian and lemon balm and sip it while you complete your prebed activity.

Practice progressive muscle relaxation. Once in bed, move through the progressive muscle relaxation exercise described on Day 2, page 78.

Give it 20 minutes. Although you've hidden your clock, if you find yourself getting anxious about the time you've spent in bed without falling asleep, get up. Turn the lamp on, read some more, or get up and go into another room and read or write in your journal until you feel sleepy again.

The Wake-Up-at-2 A.M.-and-Can't-Fall-Back-to-Sleep Insomnia

Eat for sleep. Start with a large breakfast, follow with a mid-sized lunch, and end with a light dinner, filled with tryptophan-containing foods (see Day 4 for specifics).

Cut out caffeine. Other than your one cup of morning coffee or tea, avoid food, drink, or medications containing caffeine.

Quit smoking. If you smoke, today should be the first day you try to quit. Although it's doubtful you can quit cold-turkey in one day, you can take some preliminary steps.

Make an appointment with your doctor to talk about smoking cessation aids and support groups. Try to smoke only half as many cigarettes as you normally do. Make a list of all the reasons why you want to quit, putting "a good night's sleep" at the top.

Stay sober. Avoid any alcohol with or after dinner tonight.

Review your drugs. See if any of the over-the-counter or prescription medications you're taking appear on the list of medications that can interfere with your sleep (see page 176).

Go for a long walk. After work is a good time, as it will relieve your workday stress and stretch muscles that are tight from sitting most of the day.

Darken your room. This will prevent light from waking you in the middle of the night. If you can't find blackout curtains, hang a blanket over your window. Put a nightlight in your bathroom so you don't have to turn the light on if you go to the bathroom in the middle of the night.

Don't fret. If you do wake up in the middle of the night, don't obsess about it, which can just drive up your blood pressure. Instead, try one of the relaxation/meditation techniques described on Day 2. If that doesn't work, then get up and do one of your relaxing tasks, like a crossword puzzle, cross stitch, reading, or journal-writing, until you feel sleepy again. Don't turn on any bright lights, don't eat anything, and don't try to watch TV, check your E-mail, or do any work.

The I'm-Working-the-Night-Shift-and-Can't-Fall-Asleep Insomnia

Shift workers have special problems sleeping. Shift workers trying to sleep during the day typically sleep 1.5 to 2 hours less than their night-sleeping counterparts, missing out on a significant portion of REM sleep and stage 2 sleep, resulting in "fragmented" sleep and continual exhaustion.

As one night-shift worker posted to an on-line chat room: "Help! I've been on the night shift (10 p.m.–6:30 a.m., Sun–Thurs. and sometimes Fri.) for seven years. Recently, I've gotten to where I want to sleep all the time! I've always had a problem sleeping during the day, like most shift workers, but now it seems worse. I used to sleep anywhere from four to six hours a day, and felt okay. Now, I've gotten into a routine. I go to bed around 11 a.m. I do not get up until 8:30 p.m.! I do wake up several times during this period, though. When the clock goes off, I *do not* want to get up. I feel as though I could sleep forever. I have even taken nights off just so I could stay home and sleep!"

Even when shift workers do sleep, as this shift worker described, it's interrupted sleep. The phone or doorbell rings, and lawn mowers and other outdoor sounds can be heard. You don't realize how much activity goes on in a neighborhood until you try to sleep during the day. Here are some tips:

Prepare for sleep on the way home. Wear dark sunglasses if the sun is up when you leave work so you don't reset your circadian clock too abruptly, and listen to soothing music on the ride home. As you enter your house, begin to practice your relaxation exercises (don't do this in the car), preparing your mind for sleep.

tiny movement made while sleeping. Their explorations fill more than a dozen journals devoted to sleep and the brain, yet there's so much we still don't know.

Why do we dream? Why does sleep affect our hormones so greatly? Why exactly do we sleep? If you think about it from an evolutionary perspective, it was a hardship that our ancestors had to sleep for eight hours every night, leaving themselves vulnerable to wild animals or rival tribes.

There's also the question of why we sleep so differently. Although most sleep researchers will tell you that going to bed and waking up at the same time every day is an important tool in your sleep arsenal, there are plenty of people who do just the opposite and never have any problems sleeping. There are people (like me) who can have an after-dinner cup of coffee and sleep just fine that night. There are people who follow every rule in the book for sleeping well and still wake up bleary-eyed and exhausted.

That's why it's so important that you take from the Seven-Day Sleep Program those aspects that work for you, discarding the rest. It's also important that you continue tracking your efforts in your sleep diary. Note what works and what doesn't, and every few weeks, take a look at the results and revamp your program if necessary. For sleep is not static, but as mutable as life itself. And as your life goes, so goes your sleep.

Good night, and pleasant dreams.

Five

When Something Really Is Wrong: Chronic Sleep-Related Disorders

WHEN SARAH WOKE UP IN THE MORNING, THERE WERE candy bar wrappers all over the kitchen and she had a stomachache. She also had chocolate on her face and hands. And her husband insisted that she was up eating last night. "I have no memories of doing so," says Sarah, 52. "Could he be playing a joke on me?"

Probably not. It's quite likely that Sarah is suffering from a sleep-related eating disorder, one of more than 70 serious medical conditions that can interfere with sleep. From legs that won't stop twitching, to nightmares so vivid they leave you drenched with sweat and exhausted in the morning, sleep disorders can affect not only your rest, but the rest of your life.

At least 40 million Americans each year suffer from chronic, long-term sleep disorders, and an additional 20 million experience occasional sleeping problems. These disorders and the resulting sleep deprivation interfere with work, driving, and social activities. They also account for an estimated $16 billion in medical costs each year, while the indirect costs due to lost productivity and other factors are probably much greater. The most common sleep disorders are insomnia, sleep apnea, restless legs syndrome, and narcolepsy.

Sleep Apnea

Sleep apnea, one of the most common and most dangerous sleep disorders, was first described not by a doctor, but by Charles Dickens. As the Web site talkaboutsleep (*www. talkaboutsleep.com*) notes, in *The Posthumous Papers of the Pickwick Club*, Dickens describes a very sleepy, overweight boy named Joe who snored and may have had right-sided heart failure. This led to the phrase "Pickwickian syndrome," to describe obstructive sleep apnea.

What is it? In sleep apnea, your breathing is interrupted during sleep. It typically occurs as you gain weight, or as you lose muscle tone because of aging. Both these conditions allow the windpipe to collapse during breathing when your muscles relax while you're asleep. This problem, called obstructive sleep apnea, is usually associated with loud snoring (though not everyone who snores has this disorder). Sleep apnea can also occur if the brain neurons that control breathing malfunction during sleep.

During an episode of obstructive apnea, your effort to inhale air creates suction that collapses your windpipe. This blocks the air flow for ten seconds to a minute while you struggle to breathe. When your blood oxygen level falls, your brain responds by waking you up enough to tighten the upper airway muscles and open your windpipe. You may snort or gasp, then resume snoring, all without fully awakening. This cycle may be repeated hundreds of times a night.

These frequent "awakenings" leave you continually sleepy and may lead to personality changes such as irritability or depression. One study from the University of Michigan found you don't even have to feel sleepy to have sleep apnea; just feeling low on energy during the day might be a symptom.

Sleep apnea also deprives you of oxygen, which can lead to morning headaches, a loss of interest in sex, or a decline in mental functioning. It is also linked to high blood pressure (people with moderate to severe sleep apnea are more than twice as likely to have high blood pressure), irregular heartbeats, and an increased risk of heart attacks and stroke. People with severe, untreated sleep apnea are two to three times more likely to have automobile accidents than the general population. In some high-risk individuals, sleep apnea may even lead to sudden death from respiratory arrest during sleep.

Who gets it? An estimated 18 million Americans have sleep apnea. However, few of them have had the problem diagnosed.

Diagnosis: If you have the typical features of sleep apnea, such as loud snoring, obesity, and excessive daytime sleepiness, you should be evaluated at a specialized sleep center that can perform a test called polysomnography. This test records your brain waves, heartbeat, and breathing during an entire night.

Treatment: Don't take sedatives or sleeping pills; they can prevent you from awakening enough to breathe. Mild sleep apnea can often be overcome through weight loss or simply by trying not to sleep on your back. Other people may need nasal continuous positive airway pressure (CPAP). With CPAP, you wear a mask over your nose while you sleep, and pressure from an air blower forces air through your nasal passages. This prevents your airway from closing.

Some people use dental applications that reposition the lower jaw and tongue, while others may need surgery. Common surgical procedures include removing adenoids and tonsils (especially in children), nasal polyps or other growths, or other tissue in the airway. Surgery is also performed to correct any structural deformities. These surgeries include uvulopalatopharyngoplasty and tracheostomy. Uvulopalatopharyngoplasty (UPPP) is a procedure in which excess tissue at the back of the throat (tonsils, uvula, and part of the soft palate) is removed. This procedure is successful in about 30 to 50 percent of patients. Tracheostomy is only performed in those with severe, life-threatening sleep apnea. In this procedure, the surgeon makes a small hole in your windpipe and inserts a tube into the opening. The tube stays closed during waking hours and you breathe and speak normally. But at night, it's opened so air flows directly into your lungs, bypassing any upper airway obstruction.

More recent research found that forcing your heart to beat faster during sleep with an adjustable pacemaker can also relieve sleep apnea.

Nocturnal Sleep-Related Eating Disorder (NS-RED)

What is it? In spite of its name, NS-RED is not, strictly speaking, an eating disorder. It is thought to be a type of sleep disorder in which people eat while seeming to be sound asleep. As described by the eating disorders organization, Anorexia and Related Eating Disorders, Inc. (ANRED), they may eat in bed or roam through the house and prowl the kitchen. They're not conscious during their eating episodes, which may be related to sleepwalking, and have no memories of them the next day. In fact, when they wake up and discover what they did, they're often embarrassed, ashamed, and afraid they may be losing their minds. They also tend to eat high-fat, high-sugar, comfort food that they generally don't eat while awake. Sometimes, this includes bizarre combinations of food (hot dogs dipped in peanut butter, raw bacon smeared with mayonnaise) or non-food items like soap they slice like cheese.

Victims don't eat because they're hungry, however. Researchers suspect it's due to their body's failure to react appropriately to stress. Metabolically, their bodies show a rise of melatonin and leptin (a hormone related to appetite) at night, and an increased secretion of cortisol, a hormone related to stress.

Who gets NS-RED? One to 3 percent of the general population suffer from NS-RED, but 10 to 15 percent of those with eating disorders, reports ANRED. The problem may be chronic or appear once or twice and then disappear. Many of these people are severely stressed and anxious. They're dismayed and angry at themselves for their nighttime loss of control. Many diet during the day, which may leave them hungry and vulnerable to binge eating at night when sleep weakens their control. People with NS-RED sometimes have histories of alcoholism, drug abuse, and sleep disorders other than NS-RED, such as sleepwalking, restless legs, and sleep apnea. Their sleep is fragmented, and they are often tired when they wake. The disorder, like many sleep disorders, seems to run in families, suggesting a genetic component.

Treatment. Treatment begins with a clinical interview and a night or two at a sleep-disorders center, where brain activity is monitored. Sometimes medication helps, but you shouldn't take sleeping pills. They can make matters worse by increasing confusion and clumsiness, leading to injury. Interventions that reduce stress and anxiety can also help, such as stress management classes, assertiveness training, counseling, and reducing intake of alcohol, street drugs, and caffeine.

Restless Legs Syndrome

What is it? Restless legs syndrome (RLS) is a genetically based condition whose victims have unpleasant crawling, prickling, or tingling sensations in their legs and feet and an urge to move them for relief. It's emerging as one of the most common sleep disorders, especially among older people. It leads to constant leg movement during the day and insomnia at night. In some cases, it may be linked to other conditions such as anemia, pregnancy, or diabetes. One study also found that adults with restless legs syndrome are more likely to have attention deficit hyperactivity disorder (ADHD) than those who don't have the syndrome.

Who gets it? This disorder affects as many as 12 million Americans. Many RLS patients also have a disorder known as periodic limb movement disorder or PLMD, which causes repetitive jerking movements of the limbs, especially the legs. These movements occur every 20 to 40 seconds, repeatedly awakening the victim and resulting in severely fragmented sleep. In one study, RLS and PLMD accounted for a third of the insomnia seen in patients older than age 60.

Treatment. RLS and PLMD often can be relieved by drugs that affect the neurotransmitter dopamine. Dopamine is responsible for transmitting signals within the brain, and a lack of dopamine can leave you unable to control your movements.

Narcolepsy

I once interviewed for a job with a woman who had narcolepsy. Luckily, it was a position as a medical writer, so I understood the disease. Still, it was quite disconcerting when she abruptly fell asleep during our interview, then woke a couple of minutes later as if nothing had happened.

What is it? Normally, when you're awake, your brain waves show a regular rhythm. Then, when you first fall asleep, your brain waves become slower and less regular. As we learned in Chapter 2, this sleep state is called non-rapid eye movement (NREM) sleep. After about an hour and a half of NREM sleep, the brain waves begin to show a more active pattern again, even though you're still in deep sleep. This sleep state, called rapid eye movement (REM) sleep, is when most of your dreaming occurs. In narcolepsy, the order and length of NREM and REM sleep periods are disturbed, with REM sleep occurring when you first fall asleep instead of after a period of NREM sleep. Also, some aspects of REM sleep that normally occur only during sleep—lack of muscle tone (cataplexy), sleep paralysis, and vivid dreams—occur while you're falling asleep or even while you're awake.

People with narcolepsy have frequent "sleep attacks" at various times of the day, even if they had a normal amount of nighttime sleep. These attacks last from several seconds to more than 30 minutes. Narcolepsy symptoms typically appear during adolescence, though it often takes years to obtain an accurate diagnosis. The disorder (or at least a predisposition to it) is usually hereditary, but occasionally is linked to brain damage from a head injury or neurological disease.

In 2000, scientists discovered that narcolepsy is caused by the loss of specific brain cells, resulting in a lack of a neurotransmitter called hypocretin. While hypocretin affects appetite, its connection to sleep still isn't clear. Still, this discovery should lead to new drug treatments.

Who gets it? Narcolepsy affects an estimated 250,000 Americans, but fewer than 50,000 are diagnosed. It is as widespread as Parkinson's disease or multiple sclerosis and more prevalent than cystic fibrosis, but it is less well known. Narcolepsy is often mistaken for depression, epilepsy, or the side effects of medications. It can occur in both men and women at any age, although its symptoms are usually first noticed in teenagers or young adults. There is strong evidence that narcolepsy may run in families. Eight to 12 percent of people with narcolepsy have a close relative with the disease.

Diagnosing narcolepsy: You should be checked for narcolepsy if:

- You often feel excessively and overwhelmingly sleepy during the day, even after having had a full night's sleep;
- You fall asleep when you do not intend to, such as while having dinner, talking, driving, or working;
- You collapse suddenly or your neck muscles feel too weak to hold up your head when you laugh or become angry, surprised, or shocked; or
- You find yourself briefly unable to talk or move while falling asleep or waking up.

Two tests commonly used in diagnosing narcolepsy are the polysomnogram and the multiple sleep latency test, usually performed by a sleep specialist. The polysomnogram involves continuous recording of sleep brain waves and a number of nerve and muscle functions during night-time sleep. When tested, people with narcolepsy fall asleep rapidly, enter REM sleep early, and may awaken often during the night. The polysomnogram also helps to detect other possible sleep disorders that could cause daytime sleepiness.

In a multiple sleep latency test, you're given a chance to sleep every two hours during normal wake times, while staff notes how long it takes to reach various stages of sleep. This test measures the degree of daytime sleepiness and also detects how soon REM sleep begins.

Treatment: The daytime sleepiness of narcolepsy is mainly treated with a group of drugs called central nervous system stimulants, including modafinil (Provigil), methylphenidate (Ritalin), and dextroamphetamine/methamphetamine (Dexadrine). Antidepressants and other REM-suppressing drugs, such as protriptyline (Vivactil) and fluoxetine (Prozac), are prescribed for cataplexy and other REM-sleep symptoms. Don't try to keep yourself awake with caffeine or over-the-counter drugs; they don't work.

In addition to drug therapy, an important part of treatment is scheduling short naps (10 to 15 minutes) two to three times per day to help control excessive daytime sleepiness and help you stay as alert as possible. These naps, however, aren't meant to replace nighttime sleep.

Coping With Narcolepsy

Learning as much as possible about narcolepsy and finding a support system can help patients and their families deal with the practical and emotional effects of the disease, possible occupational limitations, and situations that might cause injury. A variety of educational and other materials are available from sleep medicine or narcolepsy organizations (see Resources, page 191). There are also narcolepsy support groups.

You, your family, friends, and potential employers should know that:

- Narcolepsy is a lifelong condition that requires continuous medication.
- Although there is currently no known cure, several medications can help reduce its symptoms.
- People with narcolepsy can lead productive lives if provided with proper medical care.
- If possible, individuals with narcolepsy should avoid jobs that require driving long distances, handling hazardous equipment, or being alert for lengthy periods.
- Parents, teachers, spouses, and employers should be aware of the symptoms of narcolepsy. This will help them avoid confusing the person's behavior with laziness, hostility, rejection, or lack of interest and motivation. It will also help them provide essential support and cooperation.
- Employers can promote better working opportunities for individuals with narcolepsy by permitting special work schedules and nap breaks.

Delayed Sleep Phase Syndrome (DSPS)

What is it? With this syndrome, you go to sleep much later than most people (or even much later than when you'd like). If you try to go to sleep earlier, you have insomnia; and if you go to sleep when you want to, you have trouble waking up.

Who gets it? DSPS may affect between 5 and 10 percent of those complaining of insomnia. People with DSPS are often chronically late or absent, and consequently have problems holding day shift jobs.

Treatment: Treatment involves "resetting" your biological clock to change your sleep/wake rhythm to an earlier period using bright light exposure, medication, or chronotherapy (systemically changing your sleeping and waking times to reset your biological clock).

Advanced Sleep Phase Syndrome (ASPS)

What is it? You fall sleep earlier than the rest of the world (or earlier than you'd like). So, generally, you're excessively sleepy in the early evening, and then wake up very early in the morning.

Who gets it? This condition is very rare, occurring more often in older people.

Treatment: Treatment includes bright light and chronotherapy.

REM Sleep Behavior Disorder

What is it? Normally, you lose muscle tone during dream sleep, preventing you from physically reacting to your dreams. For reasons that are not yet understood, some people don't have this paralysis, and thus begin to move about as their dream content dictates. For instance, if you're dreaming about hitting someone, you may hit your partner.

Who gets it? This condition is very rare.

Treatment: Medications can be used to suppress dream (REM) sleep, which generally suppresses the physical activity.

Sleepwalking or Somnambulism

What is it? Like its name implies, you get out of bed before you're awake, while still in NREM sleep. Your eyes may be open, but they don't focus. If you don't wake up during the sleepwalking, you generally don't remember doing it.

Who gets it? It occurs in up to 40 percent of children, peaking at 12 years of age. Sleepwalking typically occurs in the first third of the night during deep NREM sleep (stages 3 and 4). It may also occur in adults.

Treatment. No treatment is usually required as the child usually outgrows it.

Sleep Bruxism

What is it? Sleep bruxism is the grinding or clenching of teeth during sleep. It's linked to headaches, joint discomfort and muscle aches, premature loss of teeth, and sleep disruption for both the person with bruxism and his or her partner.

Who gets it? It affects more than 8 percent of the population and is associated with other disorders such as daytime sleepiness and anxiety. It's found mostly in people aged 19 to 44, becomes less prevalent with age, and is significantly related to mental disorders, including anxiety disorders and hallucinations. About 69 percent of those with sleep bruxism related their condition to aggravation, stress, or anxiety. Daily use of alcohol, tobacco, and caffeine were also associated with the disorder.

Diagnosis: One detection method is a retainer-like device containing liquid-filled capsules. If you grind your teeth, the capsules rupture, releasing a bad-tasting liquid and waking you up, thus confirming the diagnosis.

Treatment: Treatment centers around relaxation therapies, including meditation and biofeedback training. To prevent further tooth damage, a dentist may fit you with a rubber mouth guard called an o-guard, or occlusive guard. Other devices include: oral splints; sleep alarms such as headbands and electro-monitors, which go off when you clench your jaw; and medications (although this is only temporary).

Sleep Paralysis

What is it? This condition, in which you wake up and can't move, has been around since ancient times, when it was often described as a witch or ghost sitting on your chest. Sleep paralysis strikes during the transition between REM sleep and being fully awake. It is actually a residue of the same paralysis that occurs during REM sleep, persisting for a few moments after you wake up or appearing just as you go to sleep. Generally, you can't move your body, arms, or legs. You may also have hallucinations in which you feel a presence or entity in your room. Sleep paralysis is most often associated with narcolepsy, described above. However, there are many people who experience sleep paralysis without having signs of narcolepsy.

Who gets it? Estimates vary, but one study estimated that roughly 6 percent of all people have had at least one episode of sleep paralysis, while slightly less than 1 percent have at least one episode a week. This study also found it's about five times more likely to affect those taking anti-anxiety drugs such as Xanax and and Valium. For others, the problem is often tied to sleep deprivation, a consequence of being overtired. One study found that 35 percent of subjects with isolated sleep paralysis also reported a history of waking panic attacks unrelated to the paralysis, and 16 percent met the criteria for panic disorder.

Treatment: Medication may help in severe cases, but generally, following good sleep hygiene (going to bed at the same time every day, using your bed just for sleep and sex) is the recommended treatment.

Nocturnal Paroxysmal Dystonia

What is it? This disorder is now considered to be frontal lobe epilepsy that just occurs during non-REM sleep. Victims scream and throw themselves out of bed, sometimes injuring themselves. They may make motions like they're bicycling or running across the bed.

Who gets it? The prevalence is unknown.

Treatment: It is generally treated with medication for epilepsy.

Leg Cramps

What is it? Painful sensations of muscular tightness or tension, usually in the calf, but occasionally in the foot, that occur during sleep.

Who gets it? Symptoms have been identified in up to 16 percent of healthy people, particularly following vigorous exercise. It's more common in older people, with an estimated 70 percent having leg cramps at some time. They may last for a just a few seconds or half an hour. While the cause isn't known, a lack of potassium is often associated with leg cramps.

Treatment: One meta-analysis of several studies found that quinine sulfate (200 to 300 milligrams) taken at bedtime reduced the frequency but not the severity of nocturnal leg cramps in elderly patients. Magnesium also helps (experts recommend 60 milligrams in the morning and 120 milligrams at night).

Sleep Disorders Center

Your first step in treating and diagnosing a sleep disorder is your primary care physician. He or she may then decide to refer you to a sleep disorders specialist, a doctor specially trained in diagnosing and treating sleep disorders who works at an accredited sleep center.

Once there, you'll likely have an in-depth interview with the physician, including a complete medical history. You may be asked to keep a sleep diary for several days or a week, and/or to spend one or two nights in the sleep center, where you'll have a polysomnogram, in which sensors attached to your body measure all movements, muscle activities, brain waves, and heartbeats, and your breathing and other body functions. You may also take the Multiple Sleep Latency Test to see how quickly you fall asleep, a good measure of daytime sleepiness.

To find an accredited sleep disorders center near you, go to the American Academy of Medicine Web site at *http://www.asda.org/listing.htm* and click on your state. Or call the Academy at 507-287-6006.

Six

Other Conditions That Interfere with Your Sleep

SHARLA TAYLOR RARELY GETS A GOOD NIGHT'S SLEEP. It has nothing to do with her bedroom, her breathing, or her before-bed snack. Sharla has a condition called interstitial cystitis, a chronic disease of the bladder that causes significant pain and a frequent need to go the bathroom. Consequently, she is constantly awakened either by the pain or the need to urinate. "Rarely do I sleep through the night without getting out of bed at least once," she says. "Falling back asleep is also a problem if the pain is getting to me. I usually keep the pain medicine on my nightstand so I don't have to make the trek into the kitchen. I've also found it to be true just as Bing Crosby sang: 'I count my blessings instead of sheep, then I fall asleep, counting my blessings.'"

It's amazing that, in the face of her pain and fatigue, Sharla can still be so positive. But sometimes there's just no other way to cope with the sleeplessness a medical condition can bring. Sleep and sleep-related problems play a role in a large number of human disorders and affect almost every field of medicine. Stroke and asthma attacks tend to occur more frequently during the night and early morning, perhaps due to changes in hormones, heart rate, and other characteristics associated with sleep. Sleep also affects some kinds of epilepsy in complex ways. REM sleep seems to help prevent seizures that begin in one part of the brain from spreading to other brain regions, while deep sleep may promote the spread of these seizures. Sleep deprivation also triggers seizures in people with some types of epilepsy.

In this chapter, you'll learn about the variety of medical conditions that can affect your sleep. In most cases, there are certain things you can do to improve your sleep. In many, following the Seven-Day Sleep Program should be enough. And in others, you may need your doctor's help.

Female Conditions and Sleeplessness

Sandra rarely has trouble sleeping. Rarely, that is, until the week before her period and the first couple of days of her period. Then she lies awake for hours, and when she finally falls asleep, it's a restless, dream-filled sleep from which she awakens exhausted just a few hours later, unable to fall back to sleep. "I don't understand it," she says frustrated. "It's as if this other 'being' just takes over my body." Sandra is not alone. The menstrual cycle, pregnancy, and menopause rob 56 percent of all women of sleep.

Menstruation

> *"The only time I have trouble sleeping is when I have menstrual cramps, because the pain is jarring. I have had a lot of relief from powdered magnesium/calcium in hot water. Not only does it lessen the cramping by relaxing my*

organs, but it also makes me a little drowsy, so it's all-around good."
—Mary Kittle, Allentown, Pa.

When the National Sleep Foundation conducted a special study on women and sleep problems, it found women reporting a wide range of menstrual problems affecting their sleep, including bloating, tender breasts, headaches, and cramps. On average, the poll found, sleep was disrupted for 2.5 days a month. Multiply that out for the year, and that's nearly a month of sleepless nights! Additionally, of the 73 percent of menstruating women who reported that menstrual problems affected their sleep, half identified very sleep-specific problems, ranging from feeling less refreshed to night waking and trouble falling back to sleep. As Dr. Joyce Walsleben explains in her book *A Woman's Guide to Sleep*, hormones are the most likely culprit.

During the latter part of a woman's cycle, after ovulation, progesterone levels rise. While progesterone can make you feel sleepy, it also increases your temperature, affecting your circadian rhythm and metabolic rate. Then, just before your period, when estrogen and progesterone levels drop, studies find women wake up more and have more non-REM sleep (and so wake less refreshed). Plus, if you have PMS, your sleep problems are likely worse.

Many of the steps in the Seven-Day Sleep Program will help with menstruation-related sleep disorders, as will the following:

Try calcium. Several studies have found that calcium supplements help women with premenstrual problems, including bloating, depression, and anxiety, and food cravings. In the studies, women took 1,200 milligrams of calcium carbonate in the form of Tums.

Drink water. This helps flush out your system and reduce bloating.

Consider supplements. Many of the herbal remedies described on Day 3 of the program can help with premenstrual sleep problems, and the emotional symptoms of PMS as well.

Try NSAIDs. Nonsteroidal anti-inflammatories like aspirin and ibuprofen help reduce the cramps and heavy bleeding of menstrual periods. Experts say they work best if taken daily beginning a week before your period.

Pregnancy

"My problems falling asleep relate to being nine months pregnant. Having gained an additional 43 pounds (on top of a normal weight of 108), I need seven pillows surrounding me to support my stomach, head, feet, elbows . . . My husband has to go mountain climbing to kiss me good night. I am actually looking forward to the two-hour sleep intervals when the baby arrives. At least I will be comfortable!"
　　—Marsha Shapiro, Atlanta

In the early months of pregnancy, many women do nothing but sleep. But as the pregnancy progresses, particularly in the latter stages, sleep becomes a distant memory. One study by researchers at St. Joseph's University and Delaware County Memorial Hospital, both in Pennsylvania, found that 97 percent of pregnant women fail to sleep through the night by the end of their pregnancy.

The reasons for sleep problems are many: difficulty getting comfortable, pressure on the bladder requiring frequent trips to the bathroom, anxiety about the baby and birth, vivid dreams, backaches, pain as the baby presses against the sciatic nerve, and gastric reflux as the growing uterus puts pressure on the stomach. In the study described above, nearly half the women also snored by the end of their pregnancy, and a significant portion experienced other symptoms consistent with obstructive sleep apnea, such as choking awakenings and excessive daytime sleepiness.

Pregnant women also get extremely painful leg cramps that can wake them in the middle of the night. One possible cause is decreased circulation in the legs from the pressure of the baby on blood vessels or pressure on the nerves leading to the legs. Stretching exercises, wearing support stockings during the day, and sitting with your legs up several times a day may help with cramps. As for the other pregnancy-related discomforts:

Float on pillows. Just as Marsha Shapiro did, surround yourself with pillows to buoy up your body—one between your legs, one under your stomach, one behind your back. All can help cushion your body and enable you to find a comfortable spot in bed.

Raise your bed. This may help with gastric reflux (see page 171). Put bricks or books under the legs at the head of your bed.

Kick your partner out of bed. The more room you have, the more comfortable you're likely to be. Plus, you don't have to worry about lying awake because of his snoring or movement.

Visualize a perfect birth. This will help relax you and allay your fears and anxieties.

Menopause

Once again, female hormones conspire to prevent a good night's sleep, but this time the culprit is dropping estrogen levels and the hot flashes they trigger. The flashes—really the body's way of trying to cool itself down as its temperature regulator goes haywire with fluctuating estrogen levels—leave women drenched in sweat, to the point that they often have to get up and change the bed sheets and their night clothes. In fact, the National Sleep Foundation 1998 Women and Sleep Poll found that more than 36 percent of menopausal and postmenopausal women reported hot flashes, which disrupted their sleep an average of five days a month.

To cope:

Cool off your room. Sleep with the windows open, the air conditioner on, whatever it takes to keep the room cool enough for you. If this disturbs your partner, you might want to consider asking him to sleep in another room. You need the sleep.

Cool off with cotton. Sleep in cotton. It breathes and is cooler against your skin. Also go for all-cotton sheets—no one cares if they're wrinkled.

Try herbal remedies. While the only FDA-approved medication for hot flashes is hormone replacement therapy (which has recently come under fire), several herbal remedies, such as black cohosh and dong quai, may also provide relief.

Try medication. Talk to your doctor about hormone replacement therapy or antidepressants such as Effexor, which has been found to relieve hot flashes.

Ice it down. Keep a carafe of ice water on your bedside table to sip throughout the night, though this might send you to the bathroom frequently.

Depression

"I knew something was wrong when I found myself waking up at 3 a.m., my mind racing, unable to go back to sleep. So I dragged my way through the day, then went to bed earlier and earlier at night. The worst part was that not only was I exhausted, but I just felt numb, as if all joy were missing from my life. It was like I moved in a gray fog. Luckily, I'd felt like this once before, and I called my doctor."
—Janet, 52

One of the primary signs of depression is sleeping either too much or not enough, particularly waking up early in the morning unable to fall back to sleep. People with depression often find that daytime sleepiness interferes with their daily activities, and are more likely than the general public to say they're sleeping less now as compared to five years ago, to experience insomnia, to snore, and/or to have restless legs syndrome.

If you have any of the following symptoms that have lasted for more than two weeks, you need to see your doctor. Depression is a serious—but very treatable—illness characterized by:

- An "empty" feeling, ongoing sadness, and anxiety;
- Tiredness, lack of energy;
- Loss of interest or pleasure in everyday activities, including sex;
- Sleep problems, including trouble getting to sleep, very early morning waking, and sleeping too much;
- Eating more or less than usual;

- Crying too often or too much;
- Aches and pains that don't go away when treated;
- A hard time focusing, remembering, or making decisions;
- Feeling guilty, helpless, worthless, or hopeless;
- Irritability;
- Thoughts of death or suicide; a suicide attempt.

Pain

The other day, I tried lifting some weights. I started with a ten-pound weight, but after a few repetitions, realized it was too heavy. So I picked up a lighter weight and continued with my workout. In the middle of the night, I woke in excruciating pain, trapped on my side, unable to turn over. I had to wake my husband and send him for a muscle relaxer and ibuprofen. I couldn't even turn over enough to swallow water with the pills.

According to the National Sleep Foundation, I'm not alone. The NSF reports that one out of three American adults loses more than 20 hours of sleep to pain, with 65 percent of those with pain waking up in the night, and 62 percent waking up too early because of pain. Chronic pain itself causes people to lose sleep, and the loss of sleep can magnify the pain messages that are sent to the body. It becomes a vicious cycle that is very hard to break. In fact, loss of sleep can result in pain even in people who don't have a painful condition. One study found a correlation between depriving people of non-REM stage 4 sleep and increased morning tenderness, musculoskeletal aching, and unusual fatigue—symptoms that subsided over the following recovery nights.

The most common form of pain is backache. One study found that two-thirds of those with chronic back pain have problems sleeping. Backache is followed by headaches and muscular aches and pain. Another common cause of sleep-stealing pain is arthritis, with a 1996 NSF-Gallup poll finding that 30 percent of nighttime pain sufferers experience arthritis pain at night, 60 percent of those 50 and older. Together, they lose an average of 2.2 hours of sleep—nearly 11 nights a month.

Fibromyalgia, a disorder found primarily in women that's associated with pain in muscles and tendons, has insomnia as one of its hallmarks, coupled with daytime sleepiness. Research in sleep clinics finds that people with fibromyalgia actually have abnormal EEG patterns while sleeping. They are deficient in deep, nondream sleep (slow wave sleep) and have unusually high levels of alpha activity (the normal waking rhythm of the brain) during their sleep. Many fibromyalgia sufferers say they never can get into a good, sound sleep, remaining abnormally aware of what is going on around them when they do sleep. And, as with other painful conditions, sleep deprivation seems to make the pain worse.

Heart Disease

Sleep apnea, described in Chapter 5 (see page 147), is linked to heart disease. Sleep apnea sufferers are more likely to die from heart attacks than people without apnea. If the apnea continues too long, it can lead to sudden death as the heart, overwhelmed by the lack of oxygen, just gives out. Scientists have discovered that a gene that is a marker for cardiovascular disease and Alzheimer's disease is also a marker for sleep apnea, suggesting some connection among the three. Additionally, people with congestive heart failure, a condition in which the heart can't pump out all the blood that enters its chambers, tend to have more periodic limb movements in sleep, causing them to wake more often and to suffer daytime sleepiness. People with congestive heart failure may need to sleep propped up on pillows to make breathing easier. They may also benefit from the same CPAP treatment used to treat sleep apnea (see page 149). Talk to you doctor about this.

Hypertension

About half of those with hypertension, or high blood pressure, have obstructive sleep apnea (see page 147), and about half of those with obstructive sleep apnea have hypertension. In fact, studies find that after treatment for obstructive sleep apnea, daytime and nighttime blood pressure levels decrease significantly, which may reduce the likelihood of cardiovascular complications.

Gastrointestinal Reflux Disease

About 75 percent of people with gastrointestinal reflux disease, commonly called heartburn or GERD, say their symptoms interfere with sleep and sometimes wake them up. Heartburn is a burning sensation or pain in the chest that can extend from the breastbone upward to the neck and throat, often leaving a bitter or acid taste in your mouth. The more serious form of heartburn, GERD, results when the stomach's contents, including acidic gastric juice, back up into the esophagus causing sore throat, hoarseness, chronic cough, asthma, and even the feeling of a lump in the throat. Forty percent of sufferers say the sleep they lose to heartburn makes it difficult for them to function the next day. And nearly 80 percent of those with GERD say their symptoms affect them at least once a week. Unfortunately, medication often doesn't help. Of those who use medication to control their nighttime heartburn, nearly half say current remedies do not relieve all symptoms, and more than half agree they'd try anything new to relieve heartburn at night.

There are certain steps you can take to relieve the burning:

Time your meals. Don't eat later than two to three hours before bedtime. This helps reduce stomach acid and allows your stomach to partially empty its contents. Smaller portions may also help, particularly late in the day.

Eat wisely. Avoid certain foods known to exacerbate heartburn symptoms, including chocolate, peppermint, fried and fatty foods, coffee, carbonated beverages, alcoholic beverages, citrus fruits and juices, tomato products, pepper, vinegar, ketchup, and mustard.

Chew gum. Chewing gum boosts saliva production and allows for quicker neutralization of acid in the esophagus.

Lose weight. Eating less may be the best relief for heartburn.

Stop smoking. This helps the muscle between the esophagus and stomach work better.

Raise your bed. Elevate the head of your bed four to six inches using a specially designed wedge or by putting books or bricks under the legs.

Sleep on your left side. Some studies suggest this may help with heartburn.

Cancer

Fatigue is one of the most overlooked and undertreated side effects of cancer. Yet one national survey found that 78 percent of cancer patients experience fatigue during the course of their disease—more than half experiencing it most days, if not every day. Cancer patients often have problems sleeping as a result of stress, pain, hormonal changes, or side effects (such as nausea) from their medication. Yet sleep, the time when the immune system is recharged, is particularly vital for these people. If you're a cancer patient and find you're having difficulties sleeping, talk to your doctor.

Aging

Perhaps no other age group is so bothered by sleep disorders as the elderly. People tend to sleep more lightly and for shorter time periods as they get older, although they generally need about the same amount of sleep as they needed in early adulthood. About half of all people over 65 have frequent sleeping problems, such as insomnia, and deep sleep stages in many elderly people often become very short or stop completely.

Some reports say that between 12 and 25 percent of healthy seniors have chronic insomnia. Sleep problems in older adults are so common that nearly half of all prescriptions for insomnia are written for those 65 and older.

The reasons are numerous. Physiological changes play a role, since melatonin and growth hormone production, as well as the production of other chemicals related to the sleep/wake cycle, decline as we age. Changes in body temperature also occur with age. But lifestyle changes are also to blame. Older people may be more sedentary, get less exercise and natural light, and follow a poor diet. The National Sleep Foundation notes that some researchers theorize that daytime inactivity (lack of exercise) and decreased mental stimulation leads to the "aging" of sleep. As you age, your sleep also becomes more shallow, fragmented, and variable. You may have to wake more often to go to the bathroom. Any number of factors can lead to increased sleepiness the next day.

The medications older people take may also affect their

sleep. Older people take an average of eight medications, many of them sedatives or hypnotic agents, and, as the box on page 175 indicates, medications often interfere with a good night's sleep.

Many of the diseases of aging also have sleep-related disorders associated with them, including depression, Alzheimer's disease, cardiovascular disease, pulmonary disease, and arthritis.

To maintain healthy sleep as you age:

- Stick to a regular schedule of meals.
- Try to avoid daytime naps.
- Get out every day for a walk or some other form of exercise.

Sleeping When You're Sick

As anyone who's ever had the flu knows, infectious diseases tend to make you feel sleepy. This probably happens because cytokines, chemicals your immune system produces while fighting an infection, are powerful sleep-inducing chemicals. Sleep may help your body conserve energy and other resources the immune system needs to mount an attack.

Headaches and Sleep

Many people go to sleep when they have a headache, but just as many may find that sleep causes their headache. Some people wake up with migraines. Studies find a significant link between migraines and other sleep disorders, including sleep apnea and sleepwalking. The link between migraines and sleep, notes Dr. Joyce A. Walsleben, director of the sleep disorders center at NYU School of Medicine and author of *A Woman's Guide to*

Sleep, may be the neurotransmitter serotonin, linked to both the headaches and sleep. During REM sleep, there's a significant drop in serotonin levels, which may trigger the migraine. Tension headaches often occur just when you think you should be relaxed, such as Saturday mornings, as a result of the remnants of tension left in your muscles after a stressful week.

Cluster headaches—intensely painful headaches, more common in men, that occur on one side of the head and tend to occur in "clusters" over several days or weeks, are most directly related to sleep. In fact, 75 percent of cluster headaches occur during sleep itself, usually during REM sleep, notes Dr. Walsleben. People with cluster headaches are more likely to have sleep apnea, and the lack of oxygen during the sleep apnea may be one cause of the headaches.

You may also wake up with a headache if you have slept in a strange position, put undue stress on your neck or head, have a hangover, or suffer from medical problems such as high blood pressure, allergies, or sinusitis.

Medications That Affect Sleep

Numerous medications can affect your body's ability to make and use melatonin, as well as prevent sleep in other ways. If you are taking any of these medications and find you're having trouble sleeping, talk to your doctor. He or she may be able to suggest different ways to take your medication, or may find alternatives that work just as well without enhancing your sleep problems.

Antidepressants. Some antidepressants stimulate melatonin, but others decrease it. The latter include many in the SSRI (selective serotonin reuptake inhibitors) class, including Prozac, Paxil, and Zoloft.

One study found that while Luvox increased melatonin, Celexa decreased it. Another study found that patients who took Prozac had much lower melatonin levels at night after just one week, even those who weren't depressed.

NSAIDS. Studies find nonsteroidal anti-inflammatory drugs such as ibuprofen and aspirin may reduce melatonin levels as much as 75 percent in just one night. Even acetaminophen (Tylenol) may reduce melatonin, although probably not as much as the other pain relievers.

Beta-blockers. These drugs are prescribed for various heart problems, including high blood pressure and angina. They include propranolol (Inderal), atenolol (tenormin), and metoprolol (Lopressor and Toprol). Beta-blockers have been used in laboratory animals for years to stop their production of melatonin and they have a similar, though not as dramatic, effect in humans. They can cause problems falling asleep and increase the number of nighttime awakenings.

Decongestants. Many decongestants, such as Benadryl, Actifed, and Dristan have a stimulating effect, interfering with sleep.

Bronchodilators. These medicines, used for asthma and other pulmonary diseases, can interfere with sleep.

Antihypertensives. This class of medications, used to control high blood pressure, can result in insomnia.

Corticosteroids. These medications, prescribed for asthma and allergies, often cause insomnia.

Diuretics. These drugs, used to prevent you from retaining water, can interrupt sleep if you take them at night because you need to get up to go to the bathroom.

Theophylline. One of the most common drugs used to treat asthma, this medication can disrupt sleep in some people even at low doses.

Long-acting benzodiazepines (such as Valium). These have residual sedative effects that contribute to daytime sleepiness.

Glossary of Sleep-related Terms*

Antidepressant—A class of medications most commonly used in the treatment of depression. Most antidepressants also reduce REM sleep.

Apnea—Temporary cessation of breathing. See also *Sleep Apnea*. Apnea during wakefulness is extremely rare.

Arousal—An abrupt change from sleep to wakefulness, or from a "deeper" stage of non-REM sleep to a "lighter" stage.

Awakening—The return to an awake state from any of the non-REM sleep stages or REM sleep: characterized by alpha and beta waves, voluntary eye movements, and eye blinks.

Benzodiazepines—A class of sedative medication commonly used to treat anxiety and insomnia.

Biological Clock—A term applied to the brain process that regulates 24-hour fluctuations in body temperature, hormone secretion, and a host of other bodily activities. Its most important function is to foster the daily alternation of sleep and wakefulness. The biological clock is housed in a pair of tiny bilateral brain areas called the suprachiasmatic nuclei.

Brain Waves—Spontaneous electrical activity of the brain studied by means of electroencephalography (EEG).

*Glossary used with the permission of SleepQuest, *www.sleepquest.com*

Bruxism (Toothgrinding)—Grinding one's teeth while asleep. This occurs at some time in approximately 70 percent of people; most have no noticeable side effects. However, 5 percent of victims develop symptoms such as tooth wear, jaw pain, and headaches. Episodes of grinding are more severe after stressful days.

Cardiovascular—Pertaining to the heart and blood vessels.

Cataplexy—Lack of muscle tone.

Central Nervous System (CNS)—The brain and spinal cord.

Cerebral Cortex—A part of the brain responsible for the control and integration of voluntary movement and the senses of vision, hearing, touch, etc.; it also contains centers concerned with memory, language, thought, and intellect.

Chronotherapy—Treatment of a circadian rhythm sleep disorder by systemically changing sleeping and waking times to reset your biological clock. See *Circadian Rhythms*.

Circadian Rhythms—An innate daily fluctuation of physiological or behavioral functions, including sleep/wake states, generally tied to the 24-hour daily dark/light cycle. Sometimes occurs on a 23- or 25-hour cycle when light-dark and other time cues are removed.

Continuous Positive Airway Pressure (CPAP) Machine—A medical device used to treat sleep apnea. This apparatus provides a highly effective, noninvasive therapy that eliminates blockages and prevents collapse of the upper airway by generating a prescribed level of air pressure that keeps the airway open during sleep. Air pressure is delivered through a hose to a mask that fits over the nose, or both nose and mouth. The mask is secured on the face by headgear worn over the head. The appropriate air pressure level is determined during a "CPAP titration" sleep study. The complete system consists of a programmable pressure generator, tubing, mask, and headgear. Sometimes referred to as nCPAP (nasal Continuous Positive Airway Pressure).

Deep Sleep (Delta Sleep, Slow Wave Sleep)—In sleep studies, refers to combined non-REM sleep stages 3 and 4. See *NREM Sleeps*.

Delayed Sleep Phase Syndrome—A circadian rhythm disorder in which the daily sleep/wake cycle is delayed with respect to clock time. Accordingly, the sleep phase occurs well after the conventional bedtime. Usually associated with difficulty getting up in the morning.

Delta Waves—Low-frequency, high-voltage brain waves associated with sleep stages 3 and 4. See *NREM Sleep*.

Drowsiness, Drowsy—A state of quiet wakefulness that typically occurs prior to sleep onset. If the eyes are closed, diffuse and slowed alpha activity is usually present, which then gives way to early features of stage 1 sleep. See *NREM Sleep*.

Dyssomnias—A class of sleep disorders that produce either insomnia or excessive sleepiness.

Electrodes—Small devices that transmit brain waves or other biological electrical signals from a patient to a polysomnograph machine, where the signal is amplified and displayed.

Epworth Sleepiness Scale—An index that measures the likelihood you will fall asleep during the day.

Excessive Daytime Sleepiness (EDS, Somnolence, Hypersomnia)—A subjective report of problems staying awake, accompanied by quickly falling asleep when you're sitting still.

Fatigue—A feeling of tiredness or weariness usually associated with declines in performance.

GABA (Gamma-Amniobutyric Acid)—A major neurotransmitter (chemical) in the brain, which is considered to be involved in muscle relaxation, sleep, diminished emotional reaction, and sedation. GABA is released in the greatest amount from the cerebral cortex during slow wave sleep.

Gastroesphageal Reflux Disease (GERD)—The flow of stomach acid upwards into the esophagus, which can cause arousals and disrupt sleep.

Habitual Snorers—Individuals who snore nearly every night.

Hypersomnia—Sleeping for uncharacteristically long periods of time.

Hypertension—High blood pressure.

Hypnic Myoclonia—Sudden muscle contractions that occur just before you fall asleep.

Hypoxemia—Lack of an adequate amount of oxygen in the blood.

Insomnia—Difficulty with falling asleep or staying asleep.

Jet Lag—A disturbance induced by a major rapid shift in environmental time during travel to a new time zone. Symptoms include fatigue, sleep, and impaired alertness.

Light/Dark Cycle—The periodic pattern of light (artificial or natural) alternating with darkness.

Light Sleep—A common term used to describe non-REM sleep stage 1, and sometimes, stage 2. See *NREM Sleep.*

Light Therapy—Used to treat SAD (Seasonal Affective Disorder) and other conditions. Treatment involves exposing the eyes to light of appropriate intensity and duration at the appropriate time of day to affect the timing, duration, and quality of sleep.

Melatonin—A hormone secreted by the pineal gland in the brain. Melatonin has been reported to have hypnotic properties, leading some to suggest that melatonin, which is released at night, may be an natural sleep inducer.

Multiple Sleep Latency Test (MSLT)—The standard test used to measure your daytime sleepiness by measuring how quickly you fall asleep (sleep latency). It is usually carried out in five tests at two-hour intervals. This test also helps in the diagnosis of narcolepsy. Patients with narcolepsy often go directly from wakefulness to REM sleep.

Nap—A short period of sleep generally obtained at a time separate from the daily major sleep period.

Narcolepsy—A sleep disorder characterized by excessive sleepiness, lack of muscle tone, sleep paralysis, hallucinations, and an abnormal tendency to pass directly into REM sleep from wakefulness. It was recently found to be caused by an abnormal gene in the brain.

National Commission on Sleep Disorders Research—Created by the U.S. Congress in 1990, the commission conducted a comprehensive study of the social and economic impact of sleep disorders in America, and made recommendations based on its findings to Congress in January 1993.

Neurotransmitters—Naturally occurring chemical components that transmit signals between neurons in the brain. Neurotransmitters that appear to be important in the control of sleep and wakefulness include: norepinephrine, serotonin, acetylcholine, dopamine, adrenaline, and histamine. The process of neurotransmission may be affected by other chemicals within the brain, or by natural pharmaceuticals.

Nightmare—An unpleasant and/or frightening dream that usually awakens a person from REM sleep. Occasionally called a dream anxiety attack, it is not the same as a night (sleep) terror.

Night Terrors—Also known as sleep terrors, or pavor nocturnus. Usually a disorder of childhood, characterized by a piercing scream, signs of intense fear, and unresponsiveness to other people. If awakened during a night terror, the individual is usually confused and does not remember details of the event. Night terrors are different from nightmares in that if an individual is awakened during a nightmare, he or she functions well and may have some recall of the nightmare.

Nocturnal—"Of the night"; pertains to events that happen during sleep or the hours of darkness.

Nocturnal Enuresis (Bedwetting)—The release of urine while asleep.

Noninvasive—Pertains to medical procedures that do not penetrate the skin or a body cavity.

NREM Sleep (Non-Rapid Eye Movement Sleep, Non-Rem Sleep)—All sleep stages other than REM sleep; made up of sleep stages 1 through 4. Characterized by a slowing of brain waves and some physiological functions. A state that lacks the visible rapid eye movements and twitches. See *Sleep Stages*.

Obstructive Sleep Apnea—Repetitive cessation of breathing during sleep for ten seconds or more due to complete closure (collapse) of the throat. Usually characterized by snoring, excessive daytime sleepiness, and other symptoms of fatigue. See also *Sleep Apnea*.

Periodic Limb Movement Disorder—Also known as Periodic Leg Movements of Sleep and Nocturnal Myoclonus. Characterized by periodic episodes of repetitive limb movements during sleep. The movements are often associated with a partial awakening; however, the patient is usually unaware of the limb movements or frequent sleep disruption. The number of movements may change each night.

Persistent Insomnia—Continuing insomnia that responds poorly to treatment.

Pineal Gland—A gland in the brain that secretes the hormone melatonin.

Polysomnograph—A biomedical instrument for the measurement of multiple physiological variables of sleep. It records respiratory airflow, respiratory movements, leg movements, and other parameters depending on the situation.

Pons—An area at the base of the brain that plays a role in REM sleep.

Radiofrequency (RF) Procedure (Somnoplasty)—A procedure for treating nasal obstruction, snoring, and, in some cases, sleep apnea. This procedure uses radio waves to reduce snoring and the size of the soft palate. These techniques are performed under local anesthesia as an out-patient procedure.

REM Sleep (Rapid Eye Movement Sleep)—The sleep stage in which vivid dreaming occurs; identified by the occurrence of rapid eye movements under closed eyelids. Also associated with bursts of muscular twitching, irregular breathing, irregular heart rate, and increased autonomic activity.

REM Sleep Behavior Disorder—A disorder in which the paralysis associated with REM sleep is partially or completely absent. People with this disorder are able to move their muscles and act out their dreams. The behaviors may include punching, kicking, leaping, and running from the bed.

Restless Legs Syndrome—A sleep disorder characterized by tingling, creeping, crawling, or aching sensations in the legs that tends to occur when an individual is not moving. There is an almost irresistible urge to move the legs to relieve the sensations. Inability to remain at rest can result in severe sleep disturbance.

Seasonal Affective Disorder (SAD)—A mood disorder occurring in the winter months characterized by diminished energy, hypersomnia, overeating, and depressed mood. Exposure to bright light in the morning may help alleviate or decrease symptoms.

Sedatives—Drugs that tend to calm, reduce nervousness or excitement, and foster sleep.

Serotonin—A neurotransmitter in the brain that affects mood, appetite, sexual activity, aggression, body temperature, and sleep.

Shiftwork—Working at times other than the conventional daytime hours of 9:00 a.m. to 5:00 p.m.

Sleep—The overall state in which an individual rests quiescently in a recumbent position, disengages from the environment, and becomes unresponsive to stimuli.

Sleep Apnea—Cessation of breathing for 10 or more seconds during sleep. There are two basic types of sleep apnea: *Obstructive Apnea* is caused by a closure of the air passage despite efforts to breathe; *Central Apnea* is a lack of effort to breathe. Obstructive Sleep Apnea is by far the most common type.

Sleep Architecture—The sequence and duration of each sleep stage and awakening during a sleep period.

Sleep Cycle—The progression through an orderly succession of sleep states and stages. In a healthy adult, the first cycle is always initiated by going from wakefulness to non-REM sleep. The first REM period follows the first period of non-REM sleep to complete the first sleep cycle. The two sleep states continue to alternate throughout the night with an average cycle period of about 90 minutes. A full night of normal human sleep will usually consist of four to six non-REM/REM sleep cycles. See *NREM Sleep*; *Sleep Stages*; *REM Sleep*.

Sleep Debt—The result of recurrent sleep deprivation that occurs over time, when an individual does not obtain a sufficient amount of restorative daily sleep. Sleep debt is like a monetary debt; it must be paid back at some time. The larger the sleep debt, the stronger the tendency to fall asleep. This accumulation of "lost sleep" may contribute to a decreased quality of life, the onset of related health problems, and the increased risk of injury and/or accident. See *Sleep Deprivation*.

Sleep Deprivation—An acute or chronic lack of sufficient sleep, which causes a person to feel unrefreshed when awake.

Sleep Disorders—A broad range of illnesses arising from many causes, including dysfunctional sleep mechanisms, abnormalities in physiological functions during sleep, abnormalities of the biological clock, and sleep disturbances induced by external factors.

Sleep Hygiene—Behavioral activities that either contribute to or detract from restorative sleep. Good sleep hygiene would include activities such as going to bed the same time each night, restricting caffeine, and avoiding napping during the day.

Sleep Latency—The length of time it takes to go from full wakefulness to the moment of sleep.

Sleep Log or Diary—A daily, written record of a person's sleep/wake pattern containing such information as time of retiring and arising, time in bed, estimated total sleep time, number and duration of sleep interruptions, quality of sleep, daytime naps, use of medications or caffeine beverages, and nature of waking activities.

Sleep Onset—The time from when a person attempts to fall asleep until the onset of sleep. This sleep onset normally leads to NREM stage 1 sleep, but in certain conditions, such as infancy and narcolepsy, may lead to REM stage sleep.

Sleep Paralysis—Sleep paralysis is a common part of REM sleep itself but is a disorder when it strikes outside REM sleep. Usually, people with sleep paralysis are unable to perform voluntary movements either right before they go to sleep or upon waking in the morning. One of the symptoms of narcolepsy, but also experienced by some nonnarcoleptic individuals. See *Narcolepsy*.

Sleeping Pills (Hypnotics)—Compounds that have a sedative effect and are often used to produce sleepiness. If taken frequently, you may develop a tolerance to the medication.

Sleep Spindles—Bursts of electrical activity in the brain associated with stage 2 of sleep.

Sleep Stages—Distinctive stages of sleep as demonstrated by brain patterns. See *NREM Sleep; Sleep Stages 1–4; REM Sleep*.

Sleep Stage 1 (NREM Stage 1)—A stage of NREM sleep that ensues directly from the awake state. Stage 1 normally represents 4–5 percent of total sleep.

Sleep Stage 2 (NREM Stage 2)—A stage of NREM sleep that usually accounts for 45–55 percent of total sleep time.

Sleep Stage 3 (NREM Stage 3)—A stage of NREM sleep that usually appears only in the first third of the sleep episode, and usually comprises 4–6 percent of total sleep time.

Sleep Stage 4 (NREM Stage 4)—Similar to Stage 3. Sleep walking, sleep terrors, and sleep-related enuresis (or nocturnal enuresis) episodes generally start in stage 4 or when waking up from this stage.

Sleep Talking—Talking in sleep that usually occurs in the course of temporary awakenings from NREM sleep. Can occur during REM sleep, at which time it represents a motor breakthrough of dream speech. Full consciousness is not achieved and no memory of the event remains. Sleep talking probably carries no psychological or psychiatric significance, and the content should be taken very lightly.

Sleepwalking (Somnambulism)—Arising from bed during a period when there is a simultaneous occurrence of incomplete wakefulness and NREM sleep. The eyes are usually open, but don't appear to be focusing. If victims do not awaken during the episode, they do not remember the event. An extremely common phenomenon, occurring in up to 40 percent of children, with a peak incidence at 12 years of age. Sleep walking typically occurs in the first third of the night during deep NREM sleep (stages 3 and 4).

Snoring—Sounds made during sleep caused by breathing vibrations in the pharynx. In the diagnosis of obstructive sleep apnea, snoring volume and frequency of occurrence often correlate with the severity of the condition. Snoring noise is recorded in both diagnostic sleep studies and CPAP titration studies. See *Continuous Positive Air Pressure (CPAP) Machine*.

Soft Palate—The membranous and muscular fold on the roof of the mouth that extends back from the hard palate and partially separates the oral cavity from the pharynx.

Somnoplasty—The commercial name for radiofrequency treatment of snoring, nasal obstruction, and some cases of mild sleep apnea.

Subjective Sleepiness—Feelings of sleepiness.

Thalamus—A region of the brain that plays a role in translating impulses into conscious sensations.

Tolerance—In pharmacology, refers to the reduced responsiveness to a drug's action as the result of frequent use.

Tonsils—A pair of prominent masses of tissue located opposite each other in the throat in the narrow passage from the mouth to the pharynx situated between the soft palate and the base of the tongue.

Tracheostomy—The surgical formation of an opening in the trachea made through the neck, to allow the passage of air. As a treatment for severe obstructive sleep apnea, this opening bypasses an obstruction in the airway.

Transient Insomnia—Difficulty sleeping for only a few nights.

Uvula—The small soft structure hanging from the bottom of the soft palate in the midline above the back of the tongue. It is composed of connective tissue and mucous membrane.

Uvulopalatopharyngoplasty (UPPP)—Surgical treatment for obstructive sleep apnea and snoring. This procedure is designed to open the airway behind the palate. The uvula, tonsils, and excess palatal tissue are removed. The incision is closed with sutures. The procedure is performed under general anesthesia and usually requires a one- or two-day hospital stay.

White Noise—A mixture of sound waves extending over a wide frequency range that may be used to mask unwanted noise that interferes with sleep. Also called white sound.

Withdrawal—The negative effects experienced when a person stops taking sleeping pills.

Zeitgeber—An environmental time cue that helps set your circadian rhythms. Known Zeitgebers are light and physical activity.

Resources

For General Information About Sleep

American Sleep Apnea Association
1424 K Street NW
Suite 302
Washington, DC 20005
202-293-3650
http://www.sleepapnea.org

Better Sleep Council
501 Wythe Street
Alexandria, VA 22314
703-683-8371
http://www.bettersleep.org

Narcolepsy Network
10921 Reed Hartman Highway
Suite 119
Cincinnati, OH 45242
513-891-3522
http://www.narcolepsynetwork.org

National Center for Sleep Disorders Research
Two Rockledge Center, Suite 10038
6701 Rockledge Drive, MSC 7920
Bethesda, MD 20892-7920

301-435-0199
http://www.nhlbi.nih.gov/health/public/sleep

National Heart, Lung, and Blood Institute
P.O. Box 30105
Bethesda, MD 20824-0105
(301) 592-8573
http://www.nhlbi.nih.gov

National Sleep Foundation
1522 K Street NW
Suite 500
Washington, DC 20005-1253
202-347-3471
http://www.sleepfoundation.org

Restless Legs Syndrome Foundation
819 Second Street SW
Rochester, MN 55902
507-287-6465
http://www.rls.org

Sleep Disorders Dental Society
11676 Perry Highway
Bldg. 1, Suite 1204
Wexford, PA 15090
724-935-0836
http://www.thesdds.org

Sleep-Related Web Sites

American Academy of Sleep Medicine
www.aasmnet.org

American Sleep Apnea Association
www.sleepapnea.org

Ask NOAH About: Sleep and Sleep Disorders
www.noah-health.org/english/illness/sleep/sleep.html

Brain Basics: Understanding Sleep
*www.ninds.nih.gov/health_and_medical/pubs/understanding_
sleep_brain_basic_.htm*

Canadian Sleep Society
www.css.to

InteliHealth
*http://www.intelihealth.com/IH/ihtIH/WSIHW000/24597/2
4597.html?k=navx408x24597*

MEDLINEplus Sleep Disorders
www.nlm.nih.gov/medlineplus/sleepdisorders.html

NINDS Narcolepsy Information Page
*www.ninds.nih.gov/health_and_medical/disorders/narcolep_
doc.htm*

NINDS Restless Legs Syndrome Information Page
*www.ninds.nih.gov/health_and_medical/disorders/restless_
doc.htm*

NINDS Sleep Apnea Information Page
*www.ninds.nih.gov/health_and_medical/disorders/sleep_
apnea.htm*

Restless Legs Syndrome Foundation
www.rls.org

Sleepnet.com
www.sleepnet.com

SleepQuest
www.sleepquest.com

Sleep/Wake Disorders Canada
www.swdca.org

Test Your Sleep I.Q.
www.nhlbi.nih.gov/health/public/sleep/sleep_iq.pdf

Sleep Disorders Channel
http://www.sleepdisorderchannel.net/bruxism/treatment.shtml

Books on Sleep and Sleep Disorders

Albert, Katherine A., M.D. *Get a Good Night's Sleep*, Fireside, 1997.

Alvarez, Alfred. *Night: Night Life, Night Language, Sleep and Dreams*, WW Norton & Company, 1995 (paperback 1996).

Ancoli-Israel, Sonia. *All I Want Is a Good Night's Sleep*, Mosby Year Book, 1996.

Broughton, Roger, and Robert Olgivie. *Sleep, Arousal and Performance*, Birkhauser, 1992.

Bruno, Frank Joe. *Get a Good Night's Sleep: Understand Your Sleeplessness—And Banish It Forever! (Life's Little Keys—Self-Help Strategies for a Healthier, Happier You)*, MacMillan General Reference, 1997.

Buchman, Dian Dincin, and Don R. Bensen (Editors). *The Complete Guide to Natural Sleep*, Keats Publishing, 1997.

Caldwell, J. Paul, M.D. *Sleep*, Firefly Books, 1997.

Catalano, Ellen Mohr, Charles Morin, and Wilse Webb. *Getting to Sleep: Simple Effective Methods for Falling Asleep*, New Harbinger Publishing, 1990.

Coren, Stanley. *Sleep Thieves: An Eye-Opening Exploration into the Science and Mysteries of Sleep*, Free Press, 1997.

Dement, William C., and Christopher Vaughan. *The Promise of Sleep: A Pioneer in Sleep Medicine Explains the Vital Connection Between Health, Happiness and a Good Night's Sleep*, Delacourte Press, 1999.

Dement, William C., M.D., Ph.D. *The Sleepwatchers*, Stanford Alumni Association, 1992 (second edition, Nychthemeron Press, 1996).

Dotto, Lydia. *Losing Sleep, How Your Sleeping Habits Affect Your Life*, William Morrow and Company, Inc., 1990.

Ford, Norman. *The Sleep Rx, 75 Proven Ways to Get a Good Night's Sleep*, Prentice Hall Trade, 1994.

Fritz, Roger, Ph.D. *Sleep Disorders: America's Hidden Nightmare*, National Sleep Alert, Inc., 1993.

Goldberg, Philip. *Everybody's Guide to Natural Sleep*, St. Martin's Press, 1990.

Hobson, J. Allan. *Sleep*, W.H. Freeman & Co., 1995.

Inlander, Charles B., and Cynthia K. Moran, *67 Ways to Good Sleep*, Ballantine Books (A People's Medical Society Book), 1995.

Kavey, Neil B. *50 Ways to Sleep Better*, New American Library, in association with The Sleep Disorders Center, Columbia-Presbyterian Medical Center, 1996.

Lavie, Peretz. *The Enchanted World of Sleep*, Yale University Press, 1996.

Maas, Dr. James B. *Power Sleep*, Villard/Random House, 1999.

Mitler, Elizabeth A., and Merrill M. Mitler, *101 Questions About Sleep and Dreams*, Wakefulness-Sleep Education and Research Foundation, Fourth Edition, 1993.

Moorcroft, William H. *Sleep, Dreaming and Sleep Disorders*, University Press of America, 1993.

Reite, Martin, John Ruddy, and Kim Nagel. *Concise Guide to Evaluation and Management of Sleep Disorders*, American Psychiatric Press, 1997.

Shapiro, Colin M., Ph.D. *ABC of Sleep Disorders*, BMJ Publishing Group, 1993.

Shapiro, Colin M., Ph.D. *Forensic Aspects of Sleep*, John Wiley & Sons, 1997.

Simpson, Carolyn. *Coping with Sleep Disorders*, Rosen Publishing Group, Inc., 1996.

Vafi, H., M.D., and Pamela Vafi. *How to Get a Great Night's Sleep*, Adams Media Corp., 1994.

Wong, D. Moses. *Sleep Without Drugs*, Seven Hills Book Distributors, 1994.

Zammit, Gary K., Jane A. Zanca, and Jean Zevnik (Editors). *Good Nights: How to Stop Sleep Deprivation, Overcome Insomnia, and Get the Sleep You Need*, Andrew McMeel Publishing, 1998.

Sleep-Related Aids

Water-based pillows: Chiroflow (*www.chiroflow.com*), 1-800-763-3435, and Mediflow (*www.pillowrx.com*).

Sources

ABC News. Risks of Short Sleeping. March 30, 2001.

American Academy of Otolaryngology Head and Neck Surgery. Researchers Confirm the Association Between Sleepiness and Auto Accidents. Press release, Sept. 10, 2001. Alexandria, VA

————. Treatment for Snoring Is Quick, Painless and Inexpensive. Press release, Sept. 22, 2000. Alexandria, VA.

American College of Chest Physicians. Grinding of Teeth During Sleep Associated with Other Disorders. Press release, Jan. 24, 2001. Northbrook, IL

American Academy of Neurology. ADHD More Likely in Adults with Restless Sleep Syndrome. Press release, May 7, 2001. Saint Paul, MN

The American Gastroenterological Association. Nighttime Heartburn: The Difference Between Night and Day. Press release, May 21, 2001. Bethesda, MD

American Physiological Society. Night Eating Syndrome May Be Related to the Performance of the Body—Not the Mind. Press release. Feb. 6, 2002. Bethesda, MD

Ancoli-Israel, S. What the Hebrew tradition has to say about sleep. *Psychosomatic Medicine* 63:778–787.

Aparicio-Ramon, D.V. et al. Subjective annoyance caused by environmental noise. *Journal of Environmental Pathology and Toxicology Oncology* 1993 Oct–Dec(4):237–43.

Ashjørn Mohr Drewes and Lars Arendt-Nielsen. Pain and Sleep in Medical Diseases: Interactions and Treatment Possibilities A Review. Sleep Research Online 4(2):67–76, 2001 *http://www.sro.org/2001/Drewes/67*.

Attele, A.S., J.T. Xie, and C.S. Yuan. Treatment of insomnia: an alternative approach. *Alternative Medical Review* 2000 Jun;5(3):249–59.

Balabanoy, P., and A.P. Karamanos. Central effects of AC-1 and TFG-1. *Folia Med (Plovdiv)* 1998; 40(3B Suppl 3):110–3

Berkson, Burt. *All About B vitamins*. Avery Publishing, 1998.

Better Sleep Council. Controlling the Four Factors of the Sleep Environment. Press release, Dec. 9, 1999. Alexandria, VA

————. Couples Realize Bigger *Is* Better in the Bedroom. Press release, Sept. 2001. Alexandria, VA

Bonnet, M.H., and D.L. Arand. We are chronically sleep deprived. *Sleep* 1995 Dec;18(10):908–11.

Brink, Susan. Sleepless society. *US News and World Report*, Oct. 16, 2000.

Buchbauer, G., L. Jirovetz, W. Jager, H. Dietrich, and C. Plank. Aromatherapy: evidence for sedative effects of the essential oil of lavender after inhalation. *Z Naturforsch* [C] (German Journal) Zeitschrift für Naturforschung A 1991 Nov–Dec;46(11–12):1067–72.

Carskadon, M.A. Patterns of sleep and sleepiness in adolescents. *Pediatrician* 1990;17(1):5–12.

Chamberlain, Claudine. Waking Up to Terror. ABCnews.com.

CNN. Lack of Deep Sleep Could Contribute to Weight Gain in Men. Oct. 4, 2000.

Consumer Reports. Between the sheets. Aug. 2000.

————. Mattress sets.

Coren, Stanley. *Sleep Thieves: An Eye-Opening Exploration into the Science and Mysteries of Sleep*. Free Press Paperbacks, 1996.

Dressing, H., D. Riemann, et al. Insomnia: Are valerian/balm combination of equal value to benzodiazepine? *Therapiewoche* 1992; 42:726–36.

Driver, H.S., I. Shulman, F.C. Baker, and R. Buffenstein. Energy content of the evening meal alters nocturnal body temperature but not sleep. *Physiology Behavior* 1999 Dec 1–15;68(1–2):17–23.

Dunn, C., J. Sleep, and D. Collett, Sensing an improvement: an experimental study to evaluate the use of aromatherapy, massage and periods of rest in an intensive care unit. *Journal of Advanced Nursing* 1995 Jan;21(1):34–40.

Eddy, M. and G.S. Walbroehl. Insomnia. *American Family Physician*, April 1, 1999.

Ellis, C., G. Lemmens, and D. Parkes. Pre-sleep behaviour in normal subjects. *Journal of Sleep Research* 1995 Dec;4(4):199–201.

Ford, Norman. *The Sleep RX: 75 Proven Ways to Get a Good Night's Sleep*. Prentice Hall, 1994.

Gary, K.A., A. Winokur, S.D. Douglas, S. Kapoor, L. Zaugg, and D.F. Dinges. Total sleep deprivation and the thyroid axis: effects of sleep and waking activity. *Aviat Space Environ Med*. 1996 Jun; 67(6):513–9.

Giebelhaus, V., K.P. Strohl, W. Lormes, M. Lehmann, and N. Netzer. Physical exercise as an adjunct therapy in sleep apnea—an open trial. *Sleep Breath* 2000;4(4):173–176.

Gordon, Debra L., and Julia Van Tine. *Maximum Food Power for Women*. Rodale, 2001.

Gupta, Sanjay. Is your doctor too drowsy? *Time*. March 3, 2002.

Hart, Carole. *Secrets of Serotonin*. St. Martin's Press, 1996.

Henry, Jenny. Lavender for night sedation of people with dementia. *Youandi*, Oct. 1996, 5–7.

Inlander, Charles, and Cynthia Moran. *67 Ways to Good Sleep*. Walker and Company, 1995.

Ito, T., H. Yamadera, R. Ito, H. Suzuki, K. Asayama, and S. Endo. Effects of vitamin B12 on bright light on cognitive and sleep-wake rhythm in Alzheimer-type dementia. *Psychiatry and Clinical Neuroscience* 2001 Jun;55(3):281–2.

Jamieson, Andrew Orr. Primary disorders of circadian rhythm. *Sleep Medicine Alert*, vol. 2.

King, A.C., R.F. Oman, G.S. Brassington, D.L. Bliwise, and W.L. Haskell. Moderate-intensity exercise and self-rated quality of sleep in older adults. A randomized controlled trial. *Journal of the American Medical Association* 1997 Jan 1;277(1):32–7.

Kipp, Carole. Once upon a mattress. *Delaware Woman*, March 5, 2002.

Landstrom, U., A. Knutsson, M. Lennernas, and L. Soderberg. Laboratory studies of the effects of carbohydrate consumption on wakefulness. *Nutrition and Health* 2000;13(4):213–25.

Lark, Susan. *The Chemistry of Success*. Bay Books, 2000.

Lavin, R.A., M. Pappagallo, and K.V. Kuhlemeier. Cervical pain: a comparison of three pillows. *Archives of Physical Medicine and Rehabilitation* 1997 Feb;78(2):193–8.

Lee, K.A., M.E. Zaffke, and K. Baratte-Beebe. Restless legs syndrome and sleep disturbance during pregnancy: the role of folate and iron. *Journal of Women's Health and Gender-Based Medicine* 2001 May;10(4):335–41.

Leproult, R., G. Copinschi, O. Buxton, and E. Van Cauter. Sleep loss results in an elevation of cortisol levels the next evening. *Sleep*. 1997 Oct;20(10):865–70.

Lin, Y. Acupuncture treatment for insomnia and acupuncture analgesia. *Psychiatry and Clinical Neuroscience* 1995 May;49(2):119–20.

Maas, James B. *Power Sleep*. Villard Books, 1998.

Mahowald, Mark. Assessing excessive daytime sleepiness: a complaint to be taken seriously. *Sleep Medicine Alert*, vol. IV, no. 3.

Man-Son-Hing, M., and G. Wells. Meta-analysis of efficacy of quinine for treatment of nocturnal leg cramps in elderly people. *British Medical Journal* 1995 310:13–7.

Mander, B., *et al.* 2001. Short sleep: A risk factor for insulin resistance and obesity (Abstract 183-OR). American Diabetes Association 61st Scientific Sessions. June 22–26. Philadelphia.

Mayo Clinic. Dog Tired? It Could Be Your Pooch. Press release, Feb. 15, 2002. Rochester, MN

———. Mayo Clinic Study Is First to Scientifically Document That Bed Partners Lose an Hour of Sleep Per Night Due to Snoring Spouse. Press release, Oct. 4, 1999. Rochester, MN

Medical College of Wisconsin. Sleep Disorders May Trigger Cluster Headaches. Press release, July 11, 2000. Milwaukee, WS

Methylcobalamin. *Alternative Medicine Review* 1998 Dec;3(6):461–3.

Monk, T.H., and P.C. Zee. *Circadian Rhythms, Aging and Dementia. Circadian Clocks*, vol. 12 of *Handbook of Behavioral Neurobiology*. Plenum Publishers, 2001.

Monk, T.H., and D.J. Kupfer. Circadian rhythms in healthy aging—Effects downstream from the pacemaker. *Chronobiology International*, 17(3):355–368 (2000).

Moorcroft, W.H., K.H. Kayser, and A.J. Griggs. Subjective and objective confirmation of the ability to self-awaken at a self-predetermined time without using external means. *Sleep* 1997 Jan;20(1):40–5.

Morin, C.M., C. Colecchi, J. Stone, R. Sood, and D. Brink. Behavioral and pharmacological therapies for late-life insomnia. *Journal of the American Medical Association*, vol. 281, No. 11 March 17, 1999.

National Heart, Lung and Blood Institute, National Institutes of Health. *Various fact sheets.*

National Institute of Neurological Disorders and Stroke. Bethesda, MD. Sleep: A Dynamic Activity. This is on their web site reviewed July 1, 2001

National Sleep Foundation. Public Split on Keeping Daylight Saving Time Year-Round. Press release, Oct. 25, 2001. Washington, DC

————. Scientists Find the Cause of Narcolepsy. Press release, Aug. 30, 2000. Washington, DC

————. Sleep Apnea Linked to High Blood Pressure Risk. Press release, April 2000. Washington, DC

————. Sleep Strategies for Shift Workers. Press release, revised Oct. 1999. Washington, DC

Pankhurst, F.P., and J.A. Horne. The influence of bed partners on movement during sleep. *Sleep*, 1994 Jun;17(4):308–15.

Posture Beauty Sleep Products. Worn-out Mattresses Cause Poor Sleep. Press release, no date available.

Prevention. Why exercise is the best medicine. April 2001.

Prevention Editors. *The Doctor's Book of Home Remedies for Women.* Rodale, 1997.

————. *Healing with Vitamins.* Rodale, 1997.

Reiter, Russel, and Jo Robinson. *Melatonin: Your Body's Natural Wonder Drug.* Bantam Books, 1995.

Reuters. Middle of the Night Wakening Throws Off Body Clock. April 18, 2002.

————. Migraine and Sleep Disorders Have Much in Common. Nov. 16, 1997.

————. Pacemaker is found to ease a sleeping disorder. *New York Times*, Feb. 7, 2002.

Roehrs, T., and T. Roth. Sleep, sleepiness, and alcohol use. *Alcohol Research and Health.* 2001;25(2):101–9. Review.

St. Joseph's University. Most Pregnant Women Experience Sleep Problems. Press release, Nov. 11, 2000. Philadelphia, PA

Schmitz, M., and M. Jackel. Comparative study for assessing quality of life of patients with exogenous sleep disorders (temporary sleep onset and sleep interruption disorders) treated with a hops-valerian preparation and a benzodiazepine drug. *Wien Med Wochenschr* 1998;148(13):291–8.

Sherrill, D.L., K. Kotchou, and S.F. Quan. Association of physical activity and human sleep disorders. *Archives of Internal Medicine* 1998 Sep 28; 158(17):1894–8.

Silverberg, Donald S., and Adrian Iaina. Treating obstructive sleep apnea improves. essential hypertension and quality of life. *American Family Physician*, Jan. 12, 2002.

Singh, N.A., K.M. Clements, and M.A. Fiatarone. A randomized controlled trial of the effect of exercise on sleep. *Sleep* 1997 Feb; 20(2):95–101.

Sleep News & Research. Chronic Sleep Loss Leads to 70% Higher Risk of Premature Death; May Be Factor in Recent Increase in Adult-Onset Diabetes. Press release. Jan. 28, 2002. Pleasantville, NY

Spiegel, K., R. Leproult and E. Van Cauter. Impact of sleep debt on metabolic and endocrine function. *Lancet*. 1999 Oct 23;354(9188):1435–9.

Stampi, Claudio. Leonardo's Secret: Cat Naps. *Child Development* 1998 Aug;69(4):875–87.

Stanford University. Stanford Researchers Identify Gene Associated with Sleep Apnea. Press release, June 11, 2001. Palo Alto, Ca

Ulfberg, J., and G. Fenton. Effect of Breathe Right nasal strip on snoring. *Rhinology* 1997 Jun;35(2):50–2.

University of Michigan. You Don't Have to Feel Sleepy to Have Sleep Apnea. Press release, Aug. 11, 2000. Ann Arbor, MI

University of Illinois at Urbana Champaign. Researchers Identify Molecule Crucial to Adjusting Body's Internal Clock. Press release, Dec. 6, 1999.

University of North Carolina. "Improved Snoring Treatment: Less Pain, More Gain." Press release, Sept. 15, 2002. Chapel Hill, N.C.

Veteran's Administration. Insomniacs Helped by Cognitive Therapy. Press release, April 11, 2001. Washington, DC

Walsh, J.K. and C.L. Engelhardt. The direct economic costs of insomnia in the United States for 1995. *Sleep*. 1999:22(suppl 2):S386–S393.

Washington State University. Study Indicates Majority of Patients Complaining of Insomnia Are Diagnosed with a Mental Disorder. Press release, Sept. 10, 1999.

Vitaterna, Takashashi, Turek. Overview of circadian rhythms. *Alcohol Research & Health*, vol. 25, No. 2, 2001.

Ward, Alyson. Stressed out insomniacs search for quirky sleep rituals. *Fort Worth Star Telegram*, Feb. 1, 2002.

Wellman, J.J., M. Bohannon, and G.W. Vogel. Influence of lateral motion transfer on sleep. *Journal of Perception and Motor Skills* 1999 Aug;89(1):209–17.

Wheatley, D. Kava and valerian in the treatment of stress-induced insomnia. *Phytotherapy Research* 2001 Sept., 15(6):549–51.

Whitaker, Julian. *Best Natural Remedies for Sound Sleep*. Phillips Health, 1999.

Wilkinson, R.T., and K.B. Campbell. Effects of traffic noise on quality of sleep. *Journal of the Acoustical Society of America* 1984 Feb; 75(2):468–75.

Wilkinson, T.J. H.C. Hanger, J. Elmslie, P.M. George, and R. Sainsbury. The response to treatment of subclinical thiamine deficiency in the elderly. *American Journal of Clinical Nutrition* 1997 Oct;66(4):925–8.

Wolfson, A.R. and M.A. Carskadon. Sleep schedules and daytime functioning in adolescents. *Science,* 20 July 1990, 249:244.

Youngstedt, S.D., D.F. Kripke, and J.A. Elliott. Is sleep disturbed by vigorous late-night exercise? *Medical Science & Sports Exercise* 1999 Jun;31(6):864–9.

Index